FOLK REMEDIES
THAT WORK

Other Health-Related Books by the Wilen Sisters

CHICKEN SOUP & OTHER FOLK REMEDIES

MORE CHICKEN SOUP & OTHER FOLK REMEDIES

FOLK REMEDIES
THAT WORK

A NEW, REVISED EDITION OF
LIVE AND BE WELL

JOAN WILEN
AND
LYDIA WILEN

 HarperPerennial

A Division of HarperCollinsPublishers

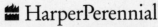

First HarperPerennial edition published 1996.

Library of Congress Cataloging-in-Publication Data

Wilen, Joan.
    Folk remedies that work / Joan Wilen and Lydia Wilen.
       p.   cm.
    Revised ed. of: Live and be well.
    Includes bibliographical references and index.
    ISBN 0-06-095164-8
    1. Alternative medicine.   2. Traditional medicine.
  I. Wilen, Lydia. II. Wilen, Joan. Live and be well.
  III. Title.
  R733.W536   1996
   615.8'8—dc20   96-5224

97 98 99 00 CC/RRD 10 9 8 7 6 5

To Our Guardian Angels
and
To All the Angels
Who Whisper in Our Ears,
Dance on Our Computer Keyboard
and
Sing in Our Hearts

$$Contents$$

Acknowledgments

Some time in the 1600s, Blaise Pascal said, "Certain authors, when they speak of their work say, 'my book.' They would be better to say 'our book,' since their writings generally contain more of other peoples' good things than their own."

There are two of us, so, naturally, we always talk in terms of "our book." But after reading Pascal's quote, the "our" has come to mean much more to us. Now when we say "our book," we refer to all the people whose "good things" are in this book; and, to the people who, *literally*, made this book possible:

The one and only—Larry Ashmead!

Special thanks for this revision to our visionary, Jason Kaufman.

Keonaona Peterson . . . and what a pleasure!

Our copy editor, Eve Potaznick, and our production editor, Mary Kurtz . . .

John Michel . . . oh, what might have been!

Elaine Markson . . . if not for her . . . and Lisa Callamaro . . . and to Pari Berg, for caring and for doing something about it.

Leona Nevler . . . for lighting the original fire. Joelle Delbourgo . . . for stoking that fire.

Ray C. Wunderlich, Jr., M.D. . . . for his wonderful input and for our peace of mind.

To name a few more, with thanks and love—Laurie Zagon, Linda Wilen, Diane, Irv, Krista & Sharron Wilen, Robert Weinstein, Gayla Snodgrass Walker, Tracy Vickery, Judy Twersky, Allen Tobias, Kathryn G. Telep, Carol Story, Barbara Stabiner, Laura Silva, Jose Silva, Rudy Shur, Priscilla Serafin, Dorothy Senerchia, Marsha Seeman, Mary Anne Kasica & Michael Scheff, Michael Samuels, Grannie Bessie Lou & Matthew Rushton, Patricia Riley, Jennifer Richards, LaVerne Reed, Kelly Neff Quattrin, Richard A. Perozzi, Joann Pelletiere, Robert Pardi, Alice Orr, Eileen Nock, Molly O'Neill, George Nider, Harvey Mirsky, Selwyn P. Miles, Bill McHugh, Elaine McDonald, Janet McCaffery, Sally Martin, Nick Malekos, Faye Hammel Levy, Ruth Landa, Kreskin, Arlen Kane, Jill Kallas, Lester Kahn, Hillary Jacobs, Eric Stephen Jacobs, Erika & Hank Holzer, Janice Herbster, Herbert A. Hartig, Lewis Harrison, Ron Hamilton, Rose Gunning, Lisa Jade Grodman, Dr. Kenneth R. Goljan, Dr. Lloyd Glauberman, Joann Furukawa, M.F.K. Fisher, Grace Ferris, Iris Featherstone, Dr. Gerald Epstein, John Ekizian, Cathy Dixon, Susie Desser, Karen Dee, Arlene Dahl, Myles Phillip Burton, Royden Brown, Treva Brown, Barbara Brennan, Eve Barth, Neil Atherton, Jamie Aromaa, and J. Walter Allen.

And to our readers . . . you have our gratitude along with our great respect for your interest in learning to take care of yourselves naturally.

FOLK REMEDIES
THAT WORK

A Wilen Sisters' Welcome

When we set out to do this book, we decided it would be an assortment of New Age as well as Age-Old remedies. The more research we did, the more we realized that in many instances, New Age *is* Age-Old, rediscovered and given New Age names.

And so, in this book, we touch on rediscovered therapies, skimming the surface in the hope of opening up a whole new healing horizon to you.

We're limited in the amount of space we can devote to any one discipline. So, if you spark to something in particular, we urge you to follow your interest. There are organizations, associations, and foundations eager to share their information. Check "Referrals" at the end of each chapter, and also the RESOURCES chapter in the book. There are wonderful books and tapes available from which to learn everything you'd ever want to know about almost anything. Check libraries, book stores, and health food stores. There are also classes, seminars, and workshops of all kinds. Not only can you broaden your knowledge, but it's a great way to meet people with shared interests. Check local schools for adult education courses, and health food stores for free publications and flyers advertising what's out there for you.

Here, then, are some of the New Age/Age-Old therapies in *Folk Remedies That Work* and brief explanations to get you started.

AFFIRMATIONS

"Pleasant words are as a honeycomb. Sweet to the soul and health to the bones." (Proverbs 16:24)

Words have power—great power.

A simple example: I had to do something for someone and I resented it. It took me away from what I wanted to be doing.

I walked around feeling angry and annoyed. All of a sudden, I seemed to turn the wrong way and I got an instant stiff neck. I became even more angry and annoyed. Then I ran into a friend on the bus. I asked to change seats with him, explaining that I had a stiff neck and couldn't look in his direction unless he sat on the other side of me. He immediately asked me what's happening in my life that was making me unhappy. Without thinking, I told him what I was doing, adding "And it's a real pain in the neck." Aha!

Our subconscious acts on our words and thoughts without discrimination. We have to be careful about what we think and say. That's why affirmations are wonderful. It's positive programming for the subconscious and, as a bonus, it makes you feel better consciously, too.

Start by assigning an appropriate affirmation to yourself. Write it down on an index card and read it over and over—at least seven times in a row, out loud if possible—time and time again throughout the day. Think about the meaning of it and when you say it, mean it. But even if you memorize it and then just say it by rote, it will make a proper impression on your subconscious.

Once you get the hang of it, and a better understanding of how deeply affected you are by your words and thoughts, you can create your own affirmations by pinpointing your physical problem and the underlying cause of it.

"The tongue of the wise is health." (Proverbs 12:18)

AROMATHERAPY

Debra Nuzzi, Master Herbalist and creator of essential oil inhalers, observes that our sense of smell is unique in that the olfactory nerve receptors are the only receptors in direct contact with the outside world. Located just beneath the brain, level with the bridge of the nose, these sensitive "hairs" pick up the fragrant molecules, transporting their message directly to the limbic system, bypassing the blood brain barrier. The limbic system is the cerebral core of emotion and memory, controlling the entire endocrine system of hormones that regulate body metabolism, stress, caloric levels, insulin balance, sexual arousal, and much more.

For aromatherapy to be effective, use only natural essential oils (not synthetic or artificial), and look for the words "true," "absolute," or "concrete" on the label. The oils are potent, so use them sparingly.

Make your own perfume by adding a few drops of your favorite essential oil to an ounce of vegetable oil or 100-proof vodka.

GEM THERAPY (CRYSTAL HEALING)

Gemologists Connie Barrett and Joyce Kaessinger, proprietors of Crystal Gardens in New York City, share with us their understanding of why and how stones can help heal.

People and stones have electromagnetic energy fields. Our energy fields are constantly shifting—going in and out of balance. Stones vibrate at a perfectly symmetrical, steady, and harmonious frequency. It's the nature of the law of the universe for everything to seek balance. When we put ourselves in direct contact with the energy of stones, we allow that energy to unblock our own energy and bring balance where there was imbalance.

The most effective way of healing yourself with a stone is to lie down on your back, head to the north (aligning your spine with the earth's axis and the earth's magnetic energy), and with the stone taped to the problem area. Stay in that position and meditate, or say an affirmation, or just relax that way for at least twenty minutes. If you can't lie down, just hold the stone and rub it. When you're not actively working with the stone, wear it or carry it with you in a pocket, pocketbook, or attaché case. A half-inch stone projects energy for up to three feet around.

Silver is a soft, flowing receptive energy; gold is considered to be very active and energizing. When stones are in jewelry, the silver or gold conductive encasements enhance the energy of the stone.

Stones are said to get you in touch with your own intuition (also known as your "higher self" or that little inner voice). To select a stone, use that intuition and choose the one that seems to call out to you. Size and cost do not count. They don't have to be big and expensive to be effective. In fact, some small stones with deep, rich colors or designs are more powerful than their muted-colored big daddies.

Traditionally, certain stones are known to be good for specific ailments. If you feel that a stone other than the suggested one is going to help you, use the one of your choice. Trust your intuition, even if it means overriding tradition. When you have a physical problem, the root of the problem may not be what the symptom is. Your higher self may direct you to the stone that's going to get to the *root* of the problem. It all gets back to: Listen to that little voice inside. If you don't want to leave any stone unturned, you may also want to follow tradition and use the stone you were attracted to, as well as the one recommended for your particular problem. That's fine. In fact, the more the merrier. There's no such thing as overdosing on stones.

After using a stone for healing, run cold water over it for fifteen seconds, allowing the negative energy to flow off the stone and down the drain. While you're at it, rinse your hands and wrists under the cold water, too.

HERBS

There are some dos, don'ts, and general rules that you should know about herbs to get full benefit from them.

• Store herbs in airtight, amber-colored (if possible), glass containers. *Glass* containers are best because herbs have volatile oils that react with plastic.

• Keep herbs away from direct sunlight and heat.

• Do not keep herbs in the refrigerator. They need to be kept in a dry place and the fridge is a moist environment.

• The consensus of opinion among herbalists is that it usually takes about a year before herbs start to lose their potency. Be sure to label and date your herbs.

• The general rule for herb preparation is to *steep* leaves and flowers and to *boil* roots, barks, and seeds. Unlike the general rule, we mostly suggest that you *steep* all herbs in just-boiled water.

- Whenever possible, use a glass or a porcelain pot to boil roots, barks, and seeds, or even just to boil water to steep the herbal leaves and flowers.

- Herbs can be powerful. Be as cautious with herbs as you know to be with prescription drugs. In most cases, *more is not better.*

- If you have a history of allergies, be especially careful about taking herbs. Start ever so slowly, allowing yourself to test for an allergic reaction. If there's any sign or symptom whatsoever, forget using it! Find a non-herbal remedy for your problem.

- *Pregnant women and children should be treated with herbs only under the supervision of an herbal health professional!* We really mean it.

- Herbs mix well with each other. If you have a couple of problems, you can prepare a tea using two or three different herbs. As herbalist Maria Treben puts it, "The medicinal herbs in God's garden know their way around the human body, and they always go to the place where they are needed."

- Always sip tea slowly rather than gulping it down. As you're sipping, you might want to give some thought to the herb's healing energy.

- An herbal poultice is used to apply soothing moist heat to an affected area. Prepare the poultice by steeping a tablespoon of an appropriate herb in hot water for five minutes. Strain out and keep the water, then wrap the herb in a piece of cheesecloth, white cloth, or unbleached muslin, and apply. As soon as the poultice is dry, dip it into the herbal water again and re-apply the moist poultice to the affected area.

- Occasionally, treat yourself to a soothing herbal bath. For at least five minutes, steep a half-cup of your favorite herb(s) in two quarts of just-boiled water. Strain, and pour the liquid into your warm bath water.

- Another way to prepare an herbal bath is to fill a cloth pouch with herbs and let it dangle under the faucet as it fills your tub with hot water.

• Tinctures are made with fresh herbs and ethyl alcohol. The alcohol draws out and preserves the healing properties of the herb. Fortunately, a wide variety of prepared herbal tinctures are available at most local health food, vitamin, and herb stores. Unless you have a problem with alcohol, tinctures are convenient to use; you can carry the little jar with you. You can put drops of tincture in water or juice, or you can take it straight— under your tongue—and it will be absorbed into the bloodstream real quick. About five drops of tincture is equivalent to one cup of herbal tea. Dosage varies according to the tincture. Check the label for the manufacturer's suggested amount.

VISUALIZATION

In the following analogy, Dr. Gerald Epstein, psychiatrist and author of *Healing Visualizations* (Bantam Books, 1989), poetically describes the way in which visualization, or mental imagery, can be used to help you heal yourself and create your own good health.

I look at our individual lives as gardens that need to be tended. We are all essentially gardeners entrusted with our own reality-gardens. As gardeners, we have special functions, primarily weeding, seeding, and, of course, harvesting.

Gardens that are full of weeds cannot be harvested properly. Weeds will overrun the seeds and prevent them from taking root and blossoming. Illness, disease, and negative beliefs are weeds that we have allowed to grow in our personal gardens. Emotions such as anxiety, depression, fear, panic, worry, and despair are also weeds. Negative beliefs and emotions are intimately connected with illness and disease. It is no surprise to anyone who recognizes the basic unity of the bodymind that researchers have found a correlation between negative emotions and lowered immunity. Similarly, positive beliefs bring us positive emotions such as humor, joy, and happiness, and researchers have

shown that positive emotions are tied in with
healthy immune responses.

Mental imagery is a technique for clearing out the
old, negative weed-beliefs and replacing them with
new, positive seed-beliefs. By becoming a gardener
of your own reality, self-healing becomes possible.

Now that you know what to expect from this book, here's
what we expect from you: We expect you to listen to your inner
voice—the one that's smart and wants the best for you and that
you sometimes ignore.

We also expect you to use common sense in terms of what
to take, and dosages. In that same commonsense category is
knowing when to go to a health professional. Please keep in
mind, neither of us has medical credentials and we're not prescribing; we're writers and we're reporting. So, before starting
any self-help treatment, consult with a health professional.

It's always fun for us to hear from our readers. If you have
anything you would like to share, or if you just want to say
"hello," here's our address:

Wilen Sisters
P. O. Box 416
Ansonia Station
New York, NY 10023-416

Thank you for your interest in our book. We send you
gratitude, love, and a big hug.

May you live and be well!
Joan and Lydia

❧ ALCOHOLISM AND ❧ SOCIAL DRINKING

ALCOHOLISM

If you have a drinking problem and don't already know the government and private agencies that offer counseling, see the end of this chapter. Meanwhile, we offer suggestions to help curb the craving, along with our prayers for your recovery.

CRAVING STOPPERS

• Angelica root or angelica leaves (available at health food stores) have glutamine, an amino acid that's said to inhibit the urge for alcohol. Make tea of the herb by pouring a cup of just-boiled water over one teaspoon of angelica. Let it steep for ten minutes. Strain, add honey and lemon to taste, and drink three cups a day.

• Chaparral is a very healing herb originally used by Native Americans. Available at health food stores in capsule form. Take one capsule after every meal. It can help detoxify the liver and can curb the craving.

• Changes in your daily diet can increase your power to resist taking a drink. Let fruit, vegetables, and whole grains take the place of white flour, sugar, and all sugar products. Fortify food with B-complex vitamins by adding wheat germ and brewer's yeast to soups, stews, and cereals.

• Suck on a whole clove (the kind used in cooking) to get rid of the urge to take a drink. It's not a pleasant thing to do, but it has been known to work.

𝒮 **Affirmation:** Whenever the thought of a drink enters your mind, repeat the following sentences over and over—
I am strong. I am brave and I have control. I am getting better and better.

SOCIAL DRINKING

Drunkenness Prevention: In the (translated) words of Greek philosopher Aristotle, "Dine well on cabbage just before starting out for a big evening." In case the Romans demand equal time, here's a quote from Cato who said, "If you wish to drink much at a banquet, before dinner dip cabbage in vinegar and eat as much as you wish. When you have dined, cut five leaves. The cabbage will make you as fit as if you had had nothing and you can drink as much as you will."

What it all seems to mean is, eat cole slaw before you imbibe and you won't get drunk.

Or: Eat ten raw almonds on an empty stomach and it is said to keep you from an inebriated state.

Sober Up: Slowly eating a small grapefruit should help you sober up.

Or, get someone to juice fresh radishes for you and slowly drink half a glass of the juice.

HANGOVERS

A dark brown taste, a burning thirst,
A head that's ready to split and burst.
It is not time for mirth and laughter—
The cold gray dawn of the morning after.
—GEORGE ADE

If you're foolish enough to drink enough to have a hangover, then you deserve it! But . . . putting our personal feelings aside, we arm you with imbibing information and guidelines, prevention methods, and symptom soothers.

INFORMATION AND GUIDELINES

• Cigarettes and booze contain the same hangover-causing ingredient, acetaldehyde. So when you drink *and* smoke, you can expect a hangover from hell!

• Eat before you drink. Drinking on a full stomach slows down the body's absorption of alcohol; the slower the absorption, the less amount of alcohol reaches the brain.

• Drink twice the volume of non-alcoholic beverages as alcoholic beverages to help avoid dehydration of your body cells.

• If we thought you were interested in technical data, we'd tell you about the manufacturing by-products called "congeners" that cause all those nasty side effects from drinking. Instead, we'll tell it to ya straight—

These are the *worst* drinks in terms of hangovers: bourbon, brandy, rum, scotch, rye, cognac, whiskey, red wine, and champagne. Speaking of champagne, any bubbly alcoholic beverage, or even booze that's mixed with a carbonated drink (gin and tonic), will get into the bloodstream much faster because of the bubbles.

These are less bad than the worst drinks in terms of hangovers: vodka, gin (without the tonic), and white wine.

• The average body burns alcohol at the rate of about an ounce an hour. Drink slowly. What's the rush? (Or is that the answer?)

• Considering that the body burns alcohol at the rate of about an ounce an hour, for each ounce of alcohol you consume it will take at least an hour before you have full driving faculties. So, if you have had four ounces of alcohol by eight P.M., you should not dare to get behind the wheel of a car until—the earliest— midnight! Let's face it, chances are you're not going to stop drinking at eight P.M. Be smart. At the *start* of the partying, assign a *non-drinking* designated driver!

• Don't keep up with a friend drink for drink. Your friend may be twice your size and can drink twice as much without facing the consequences. Use your head more than your mouth.

• For women only: If you drink right before you menstruate, when the estrogen level is low, you will get drunk faster and have more severe hangovers than during any other time of your cycle.

• Incidentally, according to researchers at the Mount Sinai Medical Center, women absorb about one-third more alcohol into their blood than men. They get drunk faster and stay that way longer.

Hangover Minimizer: Take a B-complex tablet (50 mgs) *before* you start drinking and another one *while* you're drinking. Alcohol depletes the body of B vitamins, and by replenishing them, you can almost make a hangover not happen.

Hangover Prevention: When you've finished drinking and are ready for bed, stir a tablespoon of sugar into a glass of orange juice and drink it down.

This remedy came to us from a woman who took care of an alcoholic for years. She said that it prevented him from ever having a "morning after" hangover.

The fructose in the drink helps the body burn alcohol quickly.

"Morning After" Symptom Soother: Take a quarter of a lemon and rub the juicy side on each armpit. Revolting as it seems, it works.

We recommended this remedy in our book *Chicken Soup & Other Folk Remedies.* When we handed in the manuscript for the book, the publisher gave the pages to an M.D. He reviewed all the remedies to make sure they were safe. In the margins, he wrote comments like, "this is outrageous," "it's ridiculous," and "they must be joking." The doctor wasn't much for folk remedies. That is, until he came to lemon on the armpit for easing the symptoms of a hangover. In the margin, next to this remedy he wrote, "It's the greatest! Helped get me through medical school." It was our first doctor-endorsed folk remedy.

Hangover Helper: Dehydration is one of the side effects of drinking. It's important to replenish the water lost the night before. You also need to replace the electrolytes (essential nutrients like potassium) that were *flushed* away.

Drink as much water as possible before you go to bed. In the morning, eat or drink any one, two, or three of the following:

- Tomato juice (high in fructose which speeds the body's alcohol burning process)

- Tangerine juice (also relieves dry throat)

- The liquid from banana peel that was boiled in water (also eat the banana as a source of potassium)

- Watermelon

- Ten strawberries (relieves a hangover headache)

- An apple or two (relieves a hangover headache)

- Ginger root tea (four quarter-size pieces steeped for ten minutes in just-boiled water—strain and drink—especially good for an upset stomach caused by drinking)

- Sauerkraut juice

- Cabbage soup

- Chicken soup

- Beet soup (borscht)

- Tripe soup (if you're not familiar with it and have to ask for the recipe, then believe me, you wouldn't want to have it)

- Clove soup (boil a dozen cloves in a pint of water)

- Gazpacho (for *summer* hangovers)

- A tablespoon of honey (a great source of fructose)

Symptom Soother: Add a half-teaspoon of salt to eight ounces of club soda. With a straw between your teeth—horizontally, from cheek to cheek—drink the mixture. Do not sip the salted club soda *through* the straw; the liquid should pass by it on the way to being swallowed.

Hair of the Bow-Wow: If alcoholic beverages cause a hangover, it's hard for us to believe that more of the same will relieve it. But we would be remiss if we didn't include one of the best-known "hair of the dog" remedies:

Drink one or two ounces of Fernet Branca, neat. (Not being a drinker, when I first saw the remedy written that way, I thought "neat" was instructing the tipsy reader not to dribble on himself. I bet you know it means "undiluted.")

While the internationally acclaimed Fernet Branca has an alcoholic proof of about eighty percent, it also contains some wonderful extracts: aloe, gentian, rhubarb, angelica, myrrh, camomile, saffron, and peppermint.

The Fernet Branca label says it's a "bitter stimulant to the appetite." I've been told it is bitter and that first-timers want to just belt down the ounce or two.

REFERRALS

For a referral to a local chapter of a nonprofit fellowship of men and women who share their experience, strength, and hope with each other, that they may solve their common problem and help others to recover from alcoholism, write to or call:

Alcoholics Anonymous
World Services
P.O. Box 459
Grand Central Station
New York, NY 10163
212/870-3400

For a treatment referral center, call:

National Institute on Alcohol and Drug Abuse
800/662-HELP

If you think the pain you're experiencing is really gas, but you're not sure, and you're afraid it may be your appendix, we have a simple test—

Stand up straight, bring your right knee up toward your chest, stopping at your waist. Then, quickly, jut your right leg forward as though kicking something in front of you. If you get a sharp, unbearable pain anywhere in the abdominal area, you may have an inflamed appendix. If that's the case, *get medical attention immediately!*

Note: This test is not a substitute for professional diagnosis—especially if pain persists longer than your usual gas pains have in the past.

Prevention: The *British Medical Journal* reported the findings of studies that were conducted at England's University of Southampton. It seems that by liberally lacing your diet with tomatoes and a variety of green vegetables, you may reduce the chance of having appendicitis.

It is thought that there is a particular fiber in those foods that helps prevent inflammation of the appendix.

ARTHRITIS
(RHEUMATISM)

At an awards presentation, the late great comedian Jack Benny was quoted as saying, "I don't deserve this award, but I have arthritis and I don't deserve that either."

No one deserves arthritis, yet, according to the Arthritis Foundation, over 37,000,000 Americans have this painful ailment. There are at least a hundred different forms of arthritis—some involve connective tissues, most involve inflammation of one or more joints, and just about all involve pain.

With the exception of remedies for "gout," it's hard to know what remedies will work best for which other forms of arthritis. Follow your instincts. Read through the remedies below and listen for that little voice inside to say, "Yes!" Then check with your doctor for his or her "yes."

The Remarkable Gin-Soaked Raisin Remedy:

Ingredients

1 lb. of Golden Raisins
Gin (approximately 1 pint)
Glass bowl
Glass jar with lid

Spread the golden raisins evenly on the bottom of the glass bowl, and pour enough gin over the raisins to completely cover them. Let them stay that way until all the gin is absorbed by the raisins. It takes about 6 or 7 days, depending on the humidity. (You may want to *lightly* cover the bowl with a paper towel so that dust doesn't gather.) To make sure that *all* of the raisins get gin-soaked equally, occasionally take a spoon and turn the raisins over so that all sides get to sit in the gin on the bottom of the bowl.

As soon as all the gin has been absorbed, transfer the raisins to the jar, put the lid on, and keep it closed. DO NOT REFRIGERATE. Each day, eat 9 raisins . . . EXACTLY AND ONLY 9 RAISINS A DAY! It seems easiest to eat them in the morning with breakfast.

Joe Graedon, author of *The People's Pharmacy*, asked pharmacologist Brian Thomas at Research Triangle Institute to test the gin-soaked raisins for alcohol. He found that less than 1 drop of alcohol was left in 9 raisins.

Even so . . . BE SURE TO CHECK WITH YOUR HEALTH PROFESSIONAL TO MAKE SURE THAT THIS REMEDY WILL NOT CONFLICT WITH A MEDICATION YOU MAY BE TAKING, OR PRESENT A PROBLEM FOR ANY HEALTH CHALLENGE YOU MAY HAVE, PARTICULARLY AN *IRON-OVERLOAD* CONDITION.

My friend told her parents about this remedy for their minor joint and back aches and pains. Her folks followed the instructions. One day, while the mixture was marinating, the couple were baking strudel and realized they were short of raisins. Well, there went the remedy. But it was the best strudel they ever made. Wait—that's not the end of the story! They had shared the remedy with a neighbor who is a skier and was scheduled for knee surgery. He prepared the remedy and ate it on a daily basis. When last we heard, the neighbor was pain-free and his surgery had been put off indefinitely.

Some people have had dramatic results after eating the raisins for less than a week, while it has taken others a month or two or more to feel results. As with all remedies, this doesn't work for everyone. Be consistent; eat the raisins every day. Expect a miracle . . . but have patience!

Alfalfa Helps: You may want to make this one of the first remedies you try, along with or without any of the others. Alfalfa seeds and sprouts have trace minerals that seem to be lacking in people with common kinds of arthritis. Grind alfalfa seeds (available at health food stores) in a blender or a coffee bean grinder and eat a tablespoon of the ground seeds with each meal. There are alfalfa tablets, too, but it would take fifteen to twenty tablets a day to equal the value of the ground seeds.

While you're at it, add fresh alfalfa sprouts to your meals—on sandwiches or with salads—whenever you can.

Cabbage Leaves Make Pains Leave: For relief from pain, take a few cabbage leaves and steam them for ten minutes, until they're limp. While the steamed cabbage leaves are cooling, lightly massage a little olive oil on the painful area. As soon as possible, without burning yourself, place the warm cabbage leaves on the oiled area. Cover with a heavy towel to keep in the heat. Repeat the process an hour later with new cabbage leaves.

Shark Cartilage: This is available (at health food stores, vitamin shops, and pharmacies) as a food supplement. Dr. I. William Lane, in his book, *Sharks Don't Get Cancer,* reports researchers have found that shark cartilage is successful in reducing pain in approximately 70 percent of osteoarthritis and 60 percent of rheumatoid arthritis cases.

Dr. Lane says, "Experience suggests that arthritis pain can be alleviated through ingesting 1 gram of dried shark cartilage for every 15 pounds of body weight (or one 740-to-750-milligram capsule per 11 pounds of body weight), taken daily. Investigators have found this most effective when divided into 3 equal doses, each taken about 15 minutes before a meal."

According to Dr. Lane, "If major pain relief is not noted after 30 days of continuous and correct use, the cartilage will probably not work at all with your system or problem."

Look for unadulterated 100%-pure shark cartilage such as Benefin or Cartilade. It's costly; but if it works, it's worth it.

According to Dr. Ray Wunderlich, Jr., one class of persons—children, athletes, and people with compromised circulation—should be wary of prolonged usage. Be sure to check with your health professional before starting any self-help program.

A Need for Seaweed: We Americans are not used to the taste of seaweed. If you have arthritis, it's a good idea to acquire the taste for it. It can be extremely beneficial. Start with a half-teaspoon of kelp powder (available at health food stores or oriental markets) in a cup of warm water. Drink it every night at bedtime. Gradually add kelp, in piece form, to your food—soup, stew, salad. Kelp pills are also available. Follow the directions on the label.

Hawaiian Nectar: Some nutritionists feel that pineapple's enzyme, bromelain, can help reduce joint inflammation in some arthritic conditions. Drink a glass of pineapple juice after lunch and after dinner. Fresh juice is best; second best is bottled juice without additives or preservatives.

Cat Sitting: Have a cat sit on your knees, or wherever you have arthritic pain. Just like a Chihuahua somehow supposedly chases away asthma from its owner, so is a cat supposed to rid its owner of arthritis, according to German folklore. If you have arthritis and if you have a cat . . .

Take Tea and See: Certain herb teas can help relieve pain. Our four favs are yarrow tea, willow bark tea, dandelion tea, and burdock (roots or leaves) tea. All are available at most health food stores and herb shops. Steep a heaping teaspoon in a cup of just-boiled water for ten minutes. Strain and drink two or three cups a day.

Consider eliminating coffee or anything with caffeine. Caffeine seems to heighten pain for some (not all) arthritis sufferers.

Assault with Pepper: Red, hot, and effective is cayenne pepper, named after Cayenne, the South American region where it was originally grown.

There seems to be a big payoff with this treatment, but you pay a price. The treatment takes time and patience and the pain gets worse before it gets better or disappears completely. We're reporting this remedy because we think it's well worth the effort.

Check with your doctor before starting this and do it with his/her guidance. Take one or two cayenne pepper capsules three or four times a day, every day, consistently. Remember, at first the pain will probably increase for a short while and then it will subside considerably, maybe even completely.

Celery Tonic: Celery is known to neutralize uric acid and other excess acids in one's system. On a daily basis, eat fresh celery, drink celery juice, and/or celery seed tea. The more the better . . . within reason. Oh, and keep in mind that celery is a natural diuretic, if you get my drift.

Sex Can Help You Flex: There's good news and there's more good news. The good news is that sex can relieve arthritis sufferers from pain for up to six hours at a time. The theory is that sexual stimulation increases and releases the production of cortisone. More good news is that *self-*stimulation works as well as having sex with a partner. As Woody Allen said, "I was the best I ever had."

Oily Solution: Warm a tablespoon of peanut oil, and when it's cool enough, massage your inflamed joints with the oil. Do it several times a day and give it a few days to make a difference.

Nightshades: Nightshade foods release solanine, a substance that causes waste deposits that trigger an arthritic condition. By eliminating nightshade foods from the diet, some people can eliminate all the painful symptoms of arthritis.

If you haven't already tested yourself, now is the time to do it. Do not eat any of the nightshade foods: white potatoes; eggplant; tomatoes; green, red, and yellow peppers; or tobacco. If you use canned goods or packaged products, read labels carefully and make sure none of the above foods are in them. When eating in restaurants, ask the waiter for detailed contents info on the dishes you want to order. Be diligent!

While you're at it, stay away from dairy products and chocolate.

Force yourself to follow this eating plan for a full week, even if the pain seems to worsen during the first few days. If you are intolerant of nightshade foods, you'll be happy you found out about it. You'll also be pain-free as long as you stay away from those foods.

What's Shakin'?: Restrict your salt intake. Salt causes water retention and swelling, so it stands to reason that it might put more pressure on joints and add to the pain. If you *must* use salt, add it *after* preparing food rather than during. That way, you'll need only half the amount of salt without compromising the taste. See HEALTHFUL AND HELPFUL HINTS for salt substitutes.

Garlic to the Rescue: Garlic—daily doses in any way, shape, or form—can strengthen your immune system, rid you of pain, maybe even clear up your arthritic condition—and earn you the nickname "salami breath."

Actually, if you finely mince a clove of garlic and put it in orange juice or water and drink it down without chewing the garlic bits, the smell will not stay on your breath.

Supplement the raw garlic with a good, strong garlic pill. There are many new and wonderful *odorless* garlic pills out there that, according to recent reports, are as effective as the pills that cause the smell of garlic to stay with you.

Pack Up Your Troubles: Many doctors, naturopaths, and even the healer Edgar Cayce have recommended castor oil packs for relief from arthritis pain.

Because this remedy takes some effort to do, it seems to be a kind of test of how much you really want to let go of your condition. Hmmm, that should give you something to think about. While you're thinking—

For this remedy you'll need an electric heating pad, a piece of white wool flannel cloth (or cotton flannel will do) large enough to cover the affected area four times, two pieces of soft plastic—one for under your body to protect your linens and one for the affected area, a heavy towel, and a bottle of castor oil.

Fold the flannel in four thicknesses and douse it with castor oil. Put the plastic on your bed and lie down on it. Put the oiled flannel directly on your skin, where you have the pain. Next, put the other piece of plastic on the flannel, and, starting with the heating pad on "low," place the heating pad on top of the plastic. Gradually move the dial to "medium" and then to "high," but only if you can withstand the heat. Throw the towel over the whole shebang and stay that way for an hour or two.

Once you remove the pack, take a washcloth and wash the

castor oil off your skin with a mixture of one teaspoon of baking soda in a pint of room-temperature water.

Using the same flannel cloth (dousing it with castor oil each time), do the pack four nights on—at about the same time each night—and three nights off, four nights on, and three nights off. Notice a pattern forming? Also notice how the pain subsides.

Dr. Jarvis's Old Standard: And then there's Dr. Jarvis's old standard—apple cider vinegar and honey. We keep getting letters from people telling how that New England remedy gave them a new lease on life, usually within a month.

Mix two teaspoons of *raw* honey and two teaspoons of apple cider vinegar in a glass of warm water and drink it down before each meal and at bedtime.

Morning Stiffness Prevention: Sleep in a sleeping bag. There's no need to rough it on the floor. Place the sleeping bag *on* your bed and zip yourself in for the night. Your own body heat gets evenly distributed and it seems to be much healthier than an electric blanket or a heating pad and more effective in terms of ease-of-movement in the morning.

Gem Therapy: Connie Barrett, proprietor of Crystal Gardens in New York, has had people come into the shop, look around and, with arthritic fingers, instinctively reach for a carnelian. Connie feels that just by following our instincts, we find what we need. And yes, carnelian is one of the stones for arthritis sufferers, since it represents fluidity in every way including fluidity of movement.

Another stone that's used successfully by people with arthritis is green calcite. This inexpensive stone helps release mental rigidity which, in turn, releases physical rigidity.

Clairvoyant, teacher, and author Barbara Stabiner says that when you take a bath, keep a piece of coral in the tub with you and it can help alleviate arthritic pain.

Visualization: Upon rising and at bedtime, sit up in bed (if you prefer, sit on a hard-back chair) and close your eyes for a two- to three-minute visualization.

Start by breathing out all the air in your lungs, then slowly breathing in. As you exhale, visualize a huge theater marquee with bright lights flashing the number "3" three times. Take another slow, deep breath, and as you exhale, visualize the number "2" flashing three times. Take one more deep breath, slowly, and when you exhale, see the number "1" flashing three times.

Now that you're relaxed and ready, visualize yourself walking into a space age laboratory. Look around at all the high-tech equipment. As you're looking around you spot a machine with your name on it. You walk up to it and see that it's a huge vacuum cleaner. Look at the hose. It branches out so that there are two sections of hose. Follow it to its beginning and see that the opening of each hose is in the shape of a foot. Pull up a chair, sit down, and attach each hose to the bottom of each of your feet. Now reach over and press the "ON" button. The vacuum cleaner is working. Visualize each area of your body as the vacuum cleaner pulls out all the waste products and every one of the crystallized deposits that causes the pain. Once you feel that your body is completely free of toxins, press the "OFF" button.

Slowly count from one to three. Open your eyes, stretch, and feel refreshed.

♪ **Affirmation:** Repeat this affirmation ten times, first thing in the morning, then for every person you deal with during the day, and last thing at night.

I let go of anger and replace it with understanding, compassion, and love. The love is returned and I feel very loved.

GOUT

Were it not for the gout, there might not have been an American Revolution.

Instead of attending critical sessions of the British Parliament, William Pitt was home with the gout. As a result of his absence, the Stamp Act and the Tea Tax, which led to the Boston Tea Party, were passed by Parliament. And the rest is history. The rest really *is* history.

Throughout history there have been noted gout sufferers: Benjamin Franklin, Sir Francis Bacon, Michelangelo, Dr. Samuel Johnson, Charles Darwin, and Sir Isaac Newton.

Ninety-three percent of the people with gout are men over forty-five. The seven percent of women with the problem get it after menopause.

We know who has had it and who gets it. Now what is it? Gout is a metabolic malady, caused by the inadequate processing of purines that break down, producing uric acid as a by-product. It's the uric acid that causes the problem and the pain. Eliminate foods with purines and you may eliminate the painful condition. Here's how—

AVOID:
- Meat—all meat contains high amounts of uric acid
- All organ meats—liver, sweetbreads, kidneys
- Fish—anchovies, herring, sardines (even though they're recommended for people with other forms of arthritis, they aren't good for people with gout)
- Shellfish—especially clams, scallops, and mussels
- Fried foods
- Rich foods—desserts with white flour, sugar, and cream
- Vegetables high in purine—spinach, peas, asparagus
- Consommé, broth, and gravies—all high in purines
- Mushrooms

IF YOU MUST, HAVE LIMITED AMOUNTS ONLY:

- Dried beans, lentils
- Cauliflower
- Poultry with as little fat as possible—that means no goose or duck or poultry skin
- Oatmeal
- Yeast products

You may be wondering, what does that leave? Grains, especially brown rice, nuts and seeds, fresh fruits, and most raw vegetables. Aw c'mon, be a good sport and stick strictly to the above until the pain is gone, then you can gradually add some of the foods you love.

Yarrow tea, celery seed tea, and dandelion tea can neutralize the uric acid or help flush it out of your system. Throughout each day, drink three or four cups of any one or a combination of two or three teas.

The classic gout remedy is cherries. Eat four ounces of fresh Bing cherries every day. If it's not cherry season, you can drink bottled cherry juice or buy cherry juice concentrate (available at health food stores), and have one tablespoon three times a day. You can also eat frozen, canned, or cherries in a jar. People have reported good results from these as well.

While you're at it, add strawberries to your shopping list. They, too, are excellent uric acid neutralizers.

Incidentally, both cherries and strawberries are beneficial for many other kinds of arthritis.

Cut off the kernels from three fresh ears of corn. Place the stripped corncobs in a pot and add water—twice the height of the cobs. Simmer for an hour, then pour the liquid into a bottle and keep it refrigerated. Drink a cup of corncob tea after each meal, every day, until the gout is gone.

REFERRAL

For answers to medical questions, free literature, and referrals to local chapters, call:

Arthritis Foundation
9 AM to 7 PM E.S.T.—Mon–Fri
800/283-7800

ASTHMA

An asthma attack can be caused by an allergy, an infection, stress, or any combination of them. You're the specialist when it comes to you. Pay careful attention to your patterns so you can figure out what exactly triggers an attack. That's a big step toward knowing how to control the condition. Some of these remedies may help—

If, typically, the asthma starts acting up once you're in bed, an allergy to your detergents, fabric softener, and other laundry supplies may be the cause.

Or, maybe you've gone to bed too soon after eating. Stomach acidity-backup can trigger an attack in some people. If you think you have a problem with stomach acid, be sure you don't eat right before bedtime. When you do bed down, use an extra pillow so that you're almost sitting up.

One more nighttime trouble-maker for some asthmatics is a working fireplace. If you're in a room with a wood-burning fireplace, make sure some windows are open—you don't want to be inhaling the particles released by the wood burning in the fireplace.

AT THE ONSET OF AN ASTHMA ATTACK

• Drink a couple of tablespoons of concentrated cranberry juice (available at health food stores). You can also prepare your own mixture. Boil one pound of cranberries in one pint of water until the berries are very soft. Bottle and refrigerate the mixture. At the first sign of an asthma attack, take the chill out of the cranberries and take two tablespoons of it.

- Put your hands in a basin of ice-cold water. If you feel that it's agreeing with you, let your hands soak for up to fifteen minutes.

- At the very first sign of an asthma attack, peel and finely mince a clove of garlic, add it to a tablespoon of raw honey, and swallow it down. The combination of garlic and honey can quell an attack.

Asthma Attack Prevention: Drink aloe vera juice (available at health food stores)—an ounce after every meal.

According to Dr. Isadore Rosenfeld, drinking a glass of water containing 10 to 20 drops of Tabasco sauce on a regular basis will reduce the frequency and severity of asthmatic attacks. (The same drink also eases the symptoms of chronic bronchitis and the common cold.)

Studies show that vitamin B-6 (100 to 200 mgs daily) can make a major difference in preventing asthma attacks. You can overdose on B-6, so please try this remedy with the supervision of your professional health care provider.

The combination of carrot juice and ginger works wonders for preventing attacks and also for getting rid of mucus. Prepare or buy fresh carrot juice. Grate fresh ginger root, put it in cheesecloth, and squeeze out a tablespoon of ginger juice. Add it to six ounces of carrot juice and drink it in the morning and whenever you feel congested.

Respiratory Strengthener: Start playing a wind instrument. Aside from the kazoo, the harmonica is the least expensive and the easiest to learn. Discipline yourself to practice every day for at least a half-hour. It's beneficial for all respiratory problems. The Hohner Harmonica Company sent us letters—unsolicited testimonials—they've received through the years from people whose conditions have greatly improved because of playing the harmonica. Yes, music hath charm to soothe the asthmatic chest.

Clearing Up Mucus: Fenugreek seed tea (available at health food stores) seems to clear up mucus that's part of the condition. Drink a cup of the tea first thing in the morning, after every meal, and at bedtime.

Gem Therapy: Rhodochrosite is known for relieving anxiety, relaxing the muscles of the diaphragm area, and bringing oxygen into the system—all directly related to asthma.

A five-year-old boy and his mother went into Crystal Gardens, a gem shop in New York City. The boy picked up a piece of rhodochrosite and said, "Mommy, buy me this stone." The mother told her son to put it down and wait for her outside. Then she said to Joyce Kaessinger, the proprietor, "I need something for my son. He has a terrible case of asthma." Needless to say, Joyce sold the woman the rhodochrosite stone the boy had picked out.

Joyce tells that story to emphasize the point that we should follow our instincts and go with the stones we're drawn to.

In addition to rhodochrosite, citrine is a beautiful yellow stone that's said to help quell asthma attacks.

𝒮 **Affirmation:** Repeat this affirmation ten times, first thing in the morning and each time you make a decision, no matter how insignificant the decision.

I welcome today as a day of independence. It's a choice that's right for me. I can now breathe easy.

It is estimated that seventy-five million Americans have back problems ranging from occasional discomfort to chronic back pain.

Many health professionals feel that the neuromuscular imbalance that causes most chronic back pain may be an *emotional* problem rather than a *structural* one.

Dramatic positive changes can take place when one changes his/her attitude and mental frame of mind. Studies show, for instance, that falling in love can make pain disappear.

Until you fall blissfully in love, try one or more of these substitutes: Sign up for a self-help seminar like Silva Mind Method or the Forum, or any of the many helpful courses that are available; take a yoga class; do visualizations and affirmations. There's enough out there from which to choose. Do whatever it takes to expand your thinking, enlarge your beliefs, give you a more optimistic outlook, put you in control of you, and ultimately the result will be neuromuscular balance that will eliminate your back pain.

Meanwhile, here are some suggestions that can give you relief along the way.

Nothing to Sneeze At: If you have back trouble, brace yourself when you sneeze to avoid compounding the problem. If you're standing, bend your knees a little and put one hand on a nearby table. If nothing is nearby, then place your hand on your thigh. If you're seated, put your hand on a table or on your thigh. Okay, you're ready. Achoo!

For Relief from Back Pain: Take a few cabbage leaves and steam them for ten minutes, until they're limp. While the steamed cabbage leaves are cooling, lightly massage a little olive oil on the painful area of the back. As soon as possible, without burning yourself, place the warm cabbage leaves on the oiled area. Cover with a heavy towel to keep in the heat. Repeat the process an hour later with new cabbage leaves.

White willow bark capsules (available at health food stores) contain salicylate, which is the active anti-inflammatory ingredient in aspirin. Follow the recommended dosage on the label and be sure to take the capsules right *after* meals.

Caution: *If you have ulcers or tend to get heartburn, do not try the following remedy:*

In the Orient, it is believed that soaking your feet in a big basin of hot water for twenty to thirty minutes can bring relief from back pain and spasms.

When you have the feeling that your back is about to go out, you need to take the stress off that part of your body. Gather enough books to equal about a seven-inch stack and carefully lie down on the floor. Rest your head on the books and raise your knees so that your feet are flat on the floor, about a foot apart. Put your heels as close to your *tush* as possible. Now relax that way for fifteen minutes. You might want to use this time to do a visualization and affirmations.

To stand up, roll over on your side and slowly lift yourself by letting your hands and arms do most of the work.

Yarrow tea (available at health food stores) can help back problems fade away. Add a teaspoon of yarrow in a cup of just-boiled water. Let it steep for ten minutes. Strain and drink a cup before each meal and a cup at bedtime.

Color Therapy: If you have lower back problems, blue is for you. It represents sky and water and is a soothing, anti-inflammatory color. Wear a blue shirt or blouse. Surround yourself with blue things, use blue bed linens, a blue tablecloth, a blue glass or mug. If you're willing to treat yourself to some quiet time during the day, get a blue light bulb, put it in a lamp, then completely relax under that lamp for twenty minutes. You might want to say your affirmation for part of the time.

Stay away from the red clothes in your wardrobe until your back is back to normal.

COMMON SENSE DOS AND DON'TS

• Wear comfortable low- or medium-heeled shoes. Let the shoe manufacturer wear the high heels.

• If you have to lift something heavy, bend your knees, keep your back straight, and hold that heavy something close to your body.

• Push things, don't pull them, particularly if they're big and heavy.

• Sleep on your side in the fetal position.

• Don't sleep on your stomach with your head on a pillow, unless you raise your back by putting a pillow under your stomach.

• Don't sleep on a mattress that sags in the middle. A plywood board between the mattress and box spring can prevent sagging.

• Don't cradle the telephone in the crook of your neck during long phone conversations. It can cause muscular tension all the way to your lower back.

Now we go from the sensible tips above, to one of the more outrageous remedies given to us. To ease back pain, sleep with a champagne cork under your mattress.

We're trying to decide whether or not the person who swears by this remedy was in the habit of emptying out the champagne bottle before the cork went under the mattress.

Gem Therapy: Connie Barrett, one of the proprietors of Crystal Gardens, had severe lower back pain. She went to a chiropractor, got an adjustment, and was told to come back two days later. She was doubled over and could hardly walk out of the office. It was then that Connie decided to work with stones. She used:

• Smoky Quartz (teaches pride in our physical bodies and physical existence. It's excellent for depression and fatigue).

- Aventurine (considered by many to be the best all-purpose healing stone. It is especially good for soothing the emotions and creating a feeling of balance and well-being).

- Green Tourmaline (is a stress reliever and strengthens the nervous system).

- Hematite (increases self-esteem. Grounding. Helps you to separate your emotions from those of others).

- Eilat Stone (composed of azurite, chrysocolla, malachite, and turquoise; helps us to blend the various elements of our being peacefully and harmoniously).

Intermittently, Connie meditated with the stones and kept them on her back for periods at a time. Forty-eight hours later, when she returned to the chiropractor, she was standing up straight, feeling as though she had never had a problem.

♪ **Lower Back Affirmation:** Repeat the affirmation at least twelve times, first thing in the morning, each time you handle money, and last thing at night.

I let go of fear and replace it with a secure feeling, knowing every thing I need is here for me now.

A blister is the kind of thing you get and then you don't stop touching it. You know you should, but what do you do? You touch it and touch it until it opens and causes you the pain you knew it would.

Now are you willing to leave it alone? Okay then, let the air get to it and dry it out naturally. Some say to dab on cornstarch—it may help. Then again, it may not. The secret is—

PREVENTION

• When you're going to be walking a lot and/or when wearing new shoes, grease up the areas of the feet where you're most likely to get blisters. Use petroleum jelly or any *thick* ointment to help resist a blister.

• Wear acrylic socks. They're layered, and instead of your feet absorbing the friction as you walk, the socks do it for you.

• Or: There's always lamb's wool. Ballerinas wrap it around their toes to soften the impact and to prevent blisters while on toe. Backpackers also use it for the same reasons.

Why expensive lamb's wool and not inexpensive absorbent cotton? Lamb's wool (available at some pharmacies and at dance shops) is wonderfully soft and substantial. Absorbent cotton doesn't hold together and doesn't offer adequate protection. Case closed!

• Legend has it that the plantain plant sprang from the body of a maiden sitting by the roadside, waiting for her lover to return. That is supposedly why plantains grow at the edge of the road.

Pick the leaves of this common plant (when you look at a picture of it in an herb book, you'll recognize it instantly), and put them in your shoes. They should prevent blisters. It is also said that they will dry up blisters you may already have.

❧ BLOOD PRESSURE ❧

When your blood pressure is taken, there are two numbers. They represent systolic pressure, the higher number that measures the force of the heartbeat, and diastolic pressure, the lower number that measures the pressure in the arteries when the heart is at rest.

Are you sure you have high blood pressure, or are you suffering from "white-coat apprehension"? White-coat apprehension, or fear of the doctor and nervousness at being tested for high blood pressure, quite often *raises* one's blood pressure. There are several other factors that could make it seem as though you have high blood pressure. If you're overweight and have large upper arms, make sure your doctor has the *large*-size cuff for taking your pressure. Using the wrong-size cuff can lead to an inaccurate reading. Drinking coffee right before having your blood pressure taken can also influence the reading. Studies show that the caffeine in two to three cups of coffee can raise your blood pressure up to fifteen percent within an hour.

According to a Canadian research project, one of every four people tested seemed to have high blood pressure, but when tested again and again, actually had normal pressure.

Be sure your doctor has the proper-size cuff and tests your pressure more than once during your visit—the second time after you've calmed down, and maybe even a third time because it's important to triple check. It's a good idea to have your pressure taken one day after another and, if possible, at different facilities or under different circumstances.

If, after being tested, you know that you are one of the over fifty-eight million Americans with high blood pressure, read on.

Studies show that vegetarians have lower blood pressure than meat eaters. We can go on telling you about studies that show how smoking cigarettes, drinking alcoholic beverages, and overeating can raise your blood pressure. Enough with the studies! Instead, let's concentrate on ways to lower your blood pressure.

Garlic and Onions: These "wonder drugs" have allicin, prostaglandin-A1, and selenium—compounds that help lower blood pressure. Eat raw garlic and onions every day. If they're too strong for you to take, there are garlic pills, onion pills, and garlic/onion pills—with or without the scent. Vitamin shops have a big selection. Be guided by the dosage on the label, allowing for your size and system. Or ask your health care provider to prescribe the appropriate dosage.

Best Bet Pet Quiz: What is the most popular household pet in the United States? To give you a chance to think about it, we'll continue this remedy a little further down.

Kiwi and Company: A kiwi a day helps keep high blood pressure away. The furry little fruit is rich in potassium and is a natural diuretic—two reasons people with high blood pressure should eat them as well as other foods high in potassium, such as ripe bananas, raw or steamed leafy green vegetables, oranges, potatoes with the scrubbed peel, and sunflower seeds.

Sing Hallelujah! Come On, Get Happy: University researchers have found that people's emotional states directly affect how high or low their blood pressure goes. When you're feeling happy, your systolic blood pressure goes down; when you're filled with anxiety, your diastolic pressure rises. Happy is better! And the good part is that your emotional state is entirely up to you. Abraham Lincoln summed it up best when he said, "Most people are about as happy as they make up their mind to be."

Hopeful Hawthorn(e): The hawthorne tree is a symbol of hope. Drinking hawthorne berry tea twice a day—in the morning and afternoon or evening—can *hopefully* help lower your blood pressure. Give it a few weeks to see results. Hawthorne berries (available at health food stores) come powdered, cut, or whole. Try each and decide which you prefer. They also come with or without the "e"—hawthorne or hawthorn.

Louisiana "Sole Food": This is a regional folk remedy that came to us from a woman in Louisiana, where Spanish moss trees grow. Take pieces of Spanish moss, sometimes referred to as "old man's beard," and walk around with them in your shoes. It's said to bring down the blood pressure.

Kelp Help: According to a U.S. Department of Agriculture scientist, there are fourteen elements essential to the proper metabolic functions of the body, and thirteen are known to be in kelp. Kelp (available in health food stores and oriental markets) is a powerful health-giving seaweed. It's as beneficial as it is bad-tasting. Who knows, maybe you'll like it more than I do.

Tear a portion of kelp into bite-sized pieces and let them soak in a glass of water overnight. In the morning, brace yourself and eat the kelp and drink the water. Kelp also comes in powder form and can be used in soups, stews, and salads. Kelp capsules are also available. Follow the recommended dosage on the label. It can be extremely effective in lowering blood pressure.

Best Bet Pet Answer: Okay, you've had enough time to think. What is the most popular household pet? If you said "fish," you'd be right and I'd be surprised.

Watching fish in a fish tank can lower blood pressure. Having a tank of fish, remembering to feed them, regulating the water temperature, cleaning the tank, and worrying about it all can raise blood pressure. The solution? Video Aquarium! All you need is a TV, VCR, and this relaxing tape of gently gliding fish. (See Referral at the end of the chapter.)

Avoid Being A-Salted: The first thing a doctor tells a patient with high blood pressure is to cut down or eliminate salt. See HEALTHFUL AND HELPFUL HINTS for some satisfying salt substitutes.

Aromatherapy: Dr. Alan R. Hirsch, director of the Smell and Taste Treatment and Research Foundation, says that some scents can significantly reduce blood pressure. The smell of the seashore is one, lavender is another, and the seemingly most effective is the smell of spiced apples.

High or Low Blood Pressure: Aloe vera juice (available at health food stores) is said to strengthen blood vessels and stabilize blood pressure. Drink an ounce after breakfast and an ounce after dinner.

𝒮 **Affirmation:** This is a longer-than-most affirmation. It's an important one and should be repeated at least ten times, starting first thing in the morning, and every hour that begins with a "t"—ten, twelve, two, three—and last thing at night.

I take comfort in knowing that where I am is exactly where I should be, and whatever is best for me will come to me. I love myself and I love my life.

REFERRAL

For video tapes of an aquarium or ocean waves or a fireplace and more, call:

The Video Naturals Co.
800/950-5545

For some time now, there's been lots of speculation and re-search about the long-term side effects of using anti-perspirants and deodorants that contain aluminum and zirconium.

Incidentally, an *anti-perspirant* is classified by the Food and Drug Administration as an over-the-counter *drug* because it retards the flow of perspiration. A *deodorant,* on the other hand (under the other arm?), has no physiological effect and is there-fore considered a *cosmetic.*

Until we know for sure about those side effects, you might have more peace of mind using these nonchemical *drugs*:

Baking Soda for That Odor: Baking soda is an inexpensive deodorant. Some people combine one part baking soda to two parts cornstarch or rice starch. You can also add a dried herb— one of your favorite fragrances. Sprinkle the mixture on your underarms right after a bath or shower.

Believe It or Not, Vinegar: Vinegar is effective protection against bacteria and body odor. With a cottonball, dab on either white vinegar or a solution of apple cider vinegar, each mixed with an equal amount of water. The vinegar smell will disap-pear within ten minutes.

When Smell Is Baddish, Use Radish: Juice up a few bunches of radishes. If you don't have a juice extractor, put the radishes in a food processor, then squeeze the juice through a piece of cheesecloth. Pour the juice into a jar, refrigerate it, and use it daily as an underarm deodorant.

Fennel Tea-riffic!: Fennel is known to be a deodorant that works from the inside out. Steep one teaspoon of fennel (available at health food stores) in a cup of just-boiled water. When it's cool, after at least five minutes, strain and drink. Have fennel tea in the morning and late afternoon. It should promote odorless perspiration.

Nuke With a Cuke: Cucumber can be used to wash and deodorize body parts. Cut a big succulent cuke in quarters and wash your perspired parts with it. Let your skin dry naturally. Cucumbers are rich in magnesium, which is said to be a natural deodorant.

Crystal Clear: If you prefer to *buy* a deodorant, there's the Thai Crystal Deodorant Stone (available at health food stores and pharmacies). This is a perfect example of a *New Age* product that's really *Age-Old.* For centuries, the people of Thailand have been using this natural crystal as deodorant. It's made from potassium sulfate and other mineral salts, crystallized over a period of months, then hand-shaped and smoothed. This Stone does not contain perfumes, emulsifiers, propellants, aluminum chlorohydrate, or any other harmful chemicals.

The Deodorant Stone leaves an invisible layer of protection that prevents odor-causing bacteria from forming on your body—underarms and feet, too.

One of these Stones is equivalent to about six cans of deodorant spray. That means the average person will be able to use the Stone for close to a year.

Glad Rags: Clothing can play a part in preventing or promoting odors. One hundred percent cotton is best.

Synthetic fabrics seem to stop the circulation of air, causing you to perspire more than usual. Certain synthetics—you'll know soon enough which ones they are—produce a strong, unpleasant smell as soon as you start to perspire.

If you have klutz tendencies, consider taking the supplement bone meal, available at health food stores. See to it that the bone meal provides you with somewhere in the neighborhood of 1,000 mgs of calcium a day. It doesn't prevent one from being a klutz; it just seems to fortify the bones so that if an accident occurs there will be bruises instead of broken bones.

Speed Healing: Take an oatstraw bath twice a week. Like bone meal mentioned above, oatstraw (available at health food stores or at herb shops) is high in calcium. Drink a cup or two of oatstraw tea daily.

Or: Eat a portion of dulse daily. It's a kind of seaweed—the kind that's most popular in England and Ireland. Also known as "sea lettuce," it is extremely health-giving and should be incorporated in one's diet under any circumstances, no less than when you have a broken bone. The vitamin K in dulse seems to promote the knitting of bones. Check out your health food store and try the different forms it comes in. It may take a while to get used to its strong oceanic taste, but a taste for it is worth cultivating.

Remedy to Bring Down Swelling: Get dried dandelion leaves (available at health food stores) and prepare two cups of strong tea. Strain out the leaves, use them for a poultice, and apply it to the swollen area. While the poultice is doing its stuff, drink the dandelion tea for more benefits. Do this twice a day— after breakfast and before dinner.

Gem Therapy: According to gem therapists, jade helps speed the healing process of broken bones. Put a piece of jade on the injured area and bind it in place. If there's a cast on the break, slip a couple of slender pieces of jade in the cast. When the bone is healed, turn the jade into jewelry and you'll have a pretty conversation piece.

◡ **Affirmation:** Repeat this affirmation at least twelve times, first thing in the morning, last thing at night, and during the day, before and after every conversation you have with anyone—

I am a tower of power, rebuilding my body and taking charge of my life.

BRUISES

Preventing Black-and-Blue Marks: As soon as you bruise yourself, wet the fingers of one hand and dip them in the sugar bowl. Then rigorously massage the injured area with your sugar-coated fingers. Make sure you reach the outer edges of the bruise. This will reduce the scope of the broken capillaries and prevent a black-and-blue mark from forming.

Or: Immediately after you bruise yourself, take a couple of tablespoons of arrowroot, add a little water to make a paste, and rub it on the area. When it dries and crumbles off, there should be no sign of a bruise.

Black-and-Blue Mark Remover: This is an amazing Chinese remedy for getting rid of a black-and-blue mark. For it, you need an egg and a silver dollar . . . the coin must be all silver. Hard-boil the egg and peel off the shell. Then hold the egg vertically and slip the silver dollar into the egg vertically until the edge of the coin is flush with the egg. While still warm, but cool enough not to burn the skin, place the egg with the coin on the black-and-blue mark. Leave it there for at least a half-hour while it somehow draws out the discoloration of the bruise.

When you open the egg to retrieve the coin, don't be surprised if the yolk is yukky—sort of marbleized.

Black Eye: Every couple of hours, gently massage castor oil on the delicate eye area. It is said to ease the pain, lessen the swelling, and minimize the discoloration.

Or: Get out the ice! No ice? Then use a package of frozen vegetables, or that movie cliché, a steak. Just make sure it's real cold. Find a routine that's comfortable, like on for five minutes, off for fifteen. It should numb the pain and keep down the swelling and discoloration.

Minor Bruise: This is a remedy I had occasion to use recently when I got my skin freakishly pinched in a duplicating machine tray. I rubbed the bruised area with the inside of a ripe banana peel. I kept the peel in place with an Ace bandage and left it on overnight. The next day, when I took it off, my skin was slightly pink where there otherwise would have been a black-and-blue mark. Banana skin stops the pain and speeds the healing process.

Slammed Finger or Toe: Oh, the pain! The remedy? CPR. No, not Cardiopulmonary Resuscitation. Our CPR stands for Cold, Pressure, and Raise it. As soon as possible after the slam, dunk the digit into ice or ice-cold water. This will stop the bleeding, internally as well as externally. Keep it there until the cold causes pain—not much longer than half-a-minute. Then, for thirty seconds put pressure on the finger by squeezing it, also to help stop the bleeding, but not tight enough to stop all circulation. While you're squeezing the injured finger, raise it above your head to slow the flow of blood. Repeat the entire one-minute procedure over and over—two, three, four dozen times. It may save you from pain, swelling, and a black finger-nail.

If you slam your finger or toe and you're too old to cry, but it hurts too much to laugh, then grate a medium-sized onion, mix in a tablespoon of salt, put the mixture in cheesecloth, and wrap it around the injured finger or toe. It should take the pain away.

Bruising and Swelling: Steep a heaping tablespoon of oregano in a cup of just-boiled water for ten minutes. Strain out and save the liquid, then put the moist oregano in cheesecloth and make a poultice. Place it on the bruised area. When the oregano dries up, moisten it with the warm liquid. An oregano poultice can relieve the pain and help bring down the swelling.

Or: Make a grated raw potato poultice and put it on the bruised area. Within two hours, there should be considerably less soreness.

For bruised and swollen knees, finely grate raw cabbage—enough to cover the whole knee. Wrap it securely in cheesecloth and place it on the knee. Then wrap plastic wrap around the knee, and around that, wrap a big towel. Change the cabbage every night before you go to bed. There should be great improvement by the fourth day.

Bruise Less: If every little bump, blow, or bang leaves you with a bruise, you may need more vitamin C in your diet. Take 500 mgs of vitamin C after breakfast and another 500 mgs after dinner. You should notice a difference in no time.

♪ **Affirmation:** The second you get a bruise, do whatever you can to ease the pain and prevent swelling, while repeating this affirmation over and over, at least two dozen times—

I recognize my goodness and my bright inner light. I love me.

Burns are categorized in degrees. It's easy to remember the *degree* of severity of each if you think of it this way—

• First degree burns damage the *first* layer of skin. They're minor burns that don't blister.

• Second degree burns damage the first and *second* layers of skin. They blister and can be serious. *Don't break the blisters.* It's Mother Nature's bandage. When the blisters break, there's danger of infection. If that's the case, consider professional health care.

• Third degree burns are downright serious! Obviously, they're deeper than first and second degree burns. Call for professional help immediately. Meanwhile, get the burned area under gently running cold water. If you need to *go* for help, put cold water on the burned area, then carefully cover it with the cleanest cloth available.

Now that you know what to do for second and third degree burns, here are some remedies for the minor, first degree burns—

Aloe Vera: The classic folk remedy for first degree burns is the gelatinous juice from the succulent aloe vera plant. This perennial plant is a potted first-aid kit that's easy to grow. It doesn't need direct sunlight or much water.

The aloe is inexpensive and can usually be found wherever plants are sold.

If you have an aloe plant and you happen to burn yourself, cut off the top of one of the lower leaves. Either peel the skin off the leaf to get at the gel, or squeeze out the healing gel and spread it on the burned area.

Carrots: Make a poultice of grated carrots and put it on the burn. If you prefer using fresh carrot juice, soak gauze or a white washcloth with the juice and apply it to the burn. Either one of these treatments should draw out the heat, lessen the pain, and promote healing.

Brown Paper Bag and Vinegar: Take a piece of paper from a clean brown paper bag, dip it in white vinegar, and apply it to the burn.

Mushrooms: The fungus among us can help heal a burn. Put mushroom slices on the affected area.

Radishes: Throw cleaned, cold radishes into a blender or food processor and purée them. Use the purée pulp as a poultice on the burn.

Baking Soda and Egg White: As soon as you burn yourself, mix enough baking soda with the white of an egg to make it a creamy solution. The sooner you apply it to the burn, the better chance you have of preventing it from blistering.

Burned Finger Tips: Have you ever reached for the wrong side of a plugged-in iron? Or, how often have you touched a too-hot-something in the oven? In the broiler? On the stove? Matt Rushton shared Grandma Bessie Mae's remedy with us for burned finger tips. Simply hold your ear lobe—place your thumb on the back side of the lobe and the burned finger tips on the front side of the lobe. Stay that way for one minute. It works like magic.

Oil Splatter Burn: Put a thin layer of honey on the burned area. Honey has very healing enzymes.

Hot Pepper Mouth Burning: After you've eaten hot peppers and your mouth feels like it's on fire, rinse your mouth with milk or yogurt or sour cream. It should take about seven minutes for the burning to subside. If you don't have any of the dairy products, chew a mouthful of white bread.

Why Wait Till the Last Minute?: Moisten a clean sponge, put it in a plastic bag, and keep it in your freezer. Should you burn yourself, whip out the sponge and put it on the seared spot.

♫ **Affirmation:** Repeat this affirmation over and over while treating the burn.

I am calm and cool and surrounded by healing energy.

Up to fifty percent of all Americans get canker sores and no one seems to know for sure what causes these viral infection flare-ups. Educated guesses are—

• Vitamin deficiency, specifically B-12, iron, and folic acid; vitamin C intolerance

• Excess of acid from foods like tomatoes, walnuts, and vinegar

• Food allergies from eggs, milk, cabbage, turnips, pork, coffee and tea, citrus fruits, walnuts and the like

• Emotional stress

Prevention: A fascinating experiment was conducted on people who get canker sores. Pin pricks were made in their mouths and that's where the canker sores formed—on the exact spots where the pin pricks were made.

Use a soft toothbrush to brush your teeth so that you won't scratch or pierce the areas of your mouth where canker sores form. This can help cut down your chances of getting canker sores.

Canker Sore Remedies:

• Eat an apple after every meal and let the potassium, pectin, and other healing-promoting properties clear up your canker sore in three or four days. If you don't have organic apples, then check HEALTHFUL AND HELPFUL HINTS on how to clean fruit so you can eat the peel and reap the benefits from it without any of the down sides.

• While the canker sore is caused by a *viral* infection, the pain of the actual sore is caused by a *bacterial* infection. Gently rinse your mouth with a mixture of 1 teaspoon of baking soda in ½ cup of warm water. That rinse can help neutralize the bacteria and relieve the pain.

• Students of the Bible or Scrabble players are familiar with myrrh. It's available at health food stores and some drug stores, in powder form, capsules, and in an alcohol solution (tincture). The latter seems to be most effective for canker sores. Dip a cotton swab in the tincture and dab the center of the sore with it. It may smart for a second, but after that the pain will be a thing of the past and soon the sore will be, too.

• Touch the center of the sore with a styptic pencil to speed up the healing process.

• Moisten the tip of your index finger with water. Dip it into dry mustard powder. Then hold the finger on the sore for five minutes. Do this three times a day. It's a painful treatment, but it works. The canker sore should be gone within forty-eight hours. If you let a canker sore run its normal course, it can take up to three weeks till it's gone.

Helpful Hint: If you have to put something like mustard powder on something like a canker sore, instead of using your finger to hold the powder in place, it may be easier and more efficient to put a dab of peanut butter on a little piece of bread and then put the mustard powder on the peanut butter. Herbs and spices stick to peanut butter better than to one's finger.

♫ **Affirmation:** Repeat this affirmation at least fifteen times, first thing in the morning, last thing at night, and each time a painful throb of the canker sore seems to be pounding on your heart—

I release all regrets now, and enjoy the best things in life.

When your child
is the size of a hug
and starts to come down with
some sort of bug
or any pain
or any ache,
consult with a doctor
for safety's sake.

And when the doctor
okays a cure,
go over the dosage
just to make sure,
keeping in mind
the child's weight and age,
which should be used
as a dosage gauge.

Growing a child
is as tough as can be.
You know that,
apPARENTly.

Asthma Breathing Exercise: Children who use the muscles of the shoulders and chest to breathe are not breathing in a relaxed way. Nevertheless, an asthmatic child *can* learn to do deep breathing and feel more relaxed. The following information is adapted from *Controlling Asthma,* © 1991 by the American Lung Association.

If you aren't sure how your child is breathing, ask your child to lie down with his or her back on the floor and with the knees bent, feet on the floor and arms at the side. Place a book just above the belly button and ask your child to breathe deeply a few times.

As air is taken in, the belly should swell out like a balloon if breathing is relaxed and deep. As air is exhaled, the belly should go flat. The book will move up and down with the deep breathing motions, or it may fall off. The chest should remain motionless.

If breathing is shallow, your child is filling and emptying only the top part of the lungs. By learning to fill the lungs from the bottom and by learning to exhale completely, your child should feel more relaxed and breathe more easily. The following exercise can really help.

If the doctor agrees, your child should do the exercise for five minutes every day. It can be done lying down, sitting, or standing.

Start by asking your child to put his or her hand just above the belly button to feel the motion of the breathing.

Next tell your child to think of the chest and belly area as a container for air. As your child breathes in through the nose, tell him or her to slowly fill the bottom of the container first and to keep filling until the belly feels puffed out and swollen like a balloon. The hand can feel it and will move with the motion.

Then ask your child to exhale calmly through the mouth as slowly as possible. Emphasize that the container must be completely empty and the stomach as flat as it can be before slowly inhaling again.

To complete the exercise, repeat the inhale and exhale process twelve times.

(Adult asthmatics can also benefit from this deep breathing exercise.)

Bad Dreams: If your child has nightmares and, after thorough investigation, you are absolutely convinced that the child is not suffering from any emotional or physical abuse, you might try a century-old remedy. Rub the soles of the child's feet with garlic to put an end to those bad dreams.

Bed-Wetting: The classic bed-wetting folk remedy is cinnamon sticks (available at health food stores and supermarkets). Have the child chew on a cinnamon stick throughout the day and especially around bedtime.

A teaspoon of raw honey at bedtime can help your child sleep better and wake up with a dry bed. Be sure the honey is raw and, if possible, from your area.

Warning: *Never,* never *give honey to a child under one year old. The spores can cause botulism.*

Bone meal tablets (available at health food stores) may work wonders. Give the child one tablet after every meal. As soon as the problem disappears, cut down the dosage.

Acupressure for Bed-Wetting: Got a minute? That's how long it takes to apply acupressure that can eliminate bed-wetting. With your palm facing you, look at your pinky. See the two lines that separate the two joints? Those are the acupressure points.

At bedtime, when you're about to tuck in your child, take his or her pinkies and, with your thumbnails, put pressure on each of the two lines on each hand for thirty seconds each, totaling a minute.

No-Nos for Bed-Wetters: For dinner and until bedtime, do not give carrots to the child who has a bed-wetting problem. Carrots are a diuretic that seem to have a powerful effect on bed-wetters.

Another no-no is television. According to research conducted in Japan, watching TV before going to bed, particularly watching violent shows, promotes bed-wetting. It is suggested that the child be assured some peace of mind for at least an hour before bedtime. That means no TV and no heavy metal music. How about quality time with a parent?

Chicken Pox: To soothe the sores and to promote scarless healing, let a cup of bran steep in just-boiled water until cool enough to touch. Strain out the water and put the soggy bran in cheesecloth. Tie it securely so the bran doesn't fall out and become messy. Then let the bran sit on the sores for ten seconds. Once you've patted all the sores, re-wet the bran and repeat the process. Do this several times a day. It can really help.

Or, stop the chicken pox itching and prevent scarring with pea water. Yes, that's spelled correctly. Buy half a pound of peas, shell them, put them in a pint of water, and let them boil for about five minutes. When it cools, strain out the peas and sponge down your child with the liquid.

Cleaning Stuffed Toys: A teddy bear and other cuddly creatures become home to dust mites. To kill those dust mites that can trigger allergic reactions such as asthma attacks, simply put the stuffed toy in a plastic bag and leave it in the freezer for 24 hours once a week. Explain to your child that his/her stuffed toy joined the Ice Capades and must be "on ice" every Monday or whenever.

Constipation: Aside from using the adult constipation remedies, in smaller doses of course, depending on the age and size of your child, you might also try rubbing the stomach with warm olive oil. Use a clockwise circular motion for about five minutes.

Coughs: You know when a child has a cough how the cough acts up at night, especially at bedtime? Take a piece of black cotton thread and tie it loosely around the child's neck. The coughing will stop . . . but only if you use *black* thread. What? You don't believe it? Okay, try and see for yourself.

Hiccups: Tell the child to form a gun with each of his hands. If you don't understand what we mean, it's okay, kids know how to do that. Next, tell the child to stretch out his arms and point the two guns at each other (in other words, the two index fingers should be facing one another). Finally, tell the child to slowly bring the guns together as close as they can get without touching. By the time that's done, the hiccups should be gone and forgotten.

If you don't want your children playing with *hand guns,* they can use any of the adult hiccup remedies.

Hyperactivity: Elaine McDonald and her young hyperactive son suffered through years of misery with his uncontrollable tantrums and mood swings. Elaine, not wanting her son to be heavily medicated, was desperate for an alternative. One day, the boy's pediatrician told Elaine about the Feingold Association of the United States (FAUS). It's a nonprofit organization run by volunteers and based on dietary regimens recommended by Benjamin Feingold, M.D.

Elaine learned all about it, promised her son that she would not eat anything he wasn't allowed to eat, and they started their new eating plan. Basically, synthetic foods, foods with artificial colors and flavors, foods with additives and preservatives, and all natural salicylates were eliminated.

In three days, Elaine noticed a positive change. After a week, the difference was like night and day. Her son's anti-social behavior had completely disappeared.

For more information about FAUS, call 1-800-321-3287.

Lice: It happens, and it's no reflection on the care you give your child. Get rid of the lousy lice by adding 20 drops of tea tree oil to the child's shampoo. Shampoo the hair and wait 10 minutes before thoroughly rinsing. Repeat the procedure in a week.

Minor Boo-Boos: Laura Silva, healer, international lecturer, and seminar leader for Silva Mind Method, teaches children to use their own healing energy to help themselves.

Laura has young people shake out their hands, then rub them vigorously together to feel the heat and the energy. She explains that they can project a beam of blue-white energy from their right hand and collect it in their left hand. The right hand is the projector; the left hand is the collector.

When a child has a minor injury, they should shake out their hands, rub them together, and put them over—close, but not touching—the hurt area. Then they should imagine the right hand projecting a beam of blue-white energy and the left hand collecting it as the hurt goes away and they feel better and better.

P.S. It works.

P.P.S. Adults can do this too.

Swallowing a Coin: If your child swallowed a coin and you are sure it's not obstructing his breathing, quick, prepare boiled sweet potatoes and have your child eat a substantial portion. The sweet potatoes can coat the coin, making it easier to "make change."

Saving a Tooth: If your child's permanent tooth is knocked out, put the tooth in a container of milk and take it, along with your child, to the dentist. If you act fast and have a skilled dentist, (s)he may be able to save the tooth.

Upset Stomach: Add the white of an egg to a cup of water. Stir it for several minutes, then strain it through cheesecloth and have the child drink it slowly. It's an old remedy that's been known to settle the stomach.

Warts: Take a piece of tracing paper, put it on the child's wart, and with a pencil, trace the wart. Take your child and the tracing paper into the bathroom. Then make sure you impress upon the child that *only Mommy or Daddy should do this.* While (s)he watches, burn the tracing paper and flush away the ashes. In about a week, the wart will disappear.

CHOKING

The universal sign for a person to use when choking is grasping the neck between the thumb and index finger of one hand. If you're with someone who is choking but doesn't know the sign, you should know—

HOW TO RECOGNIZE WHEN SOMEONE IS CHOKING

• Suddenly the person cannot speak, breathe, or cough.

• The person may frantically toss his head and, in a panic, get up quickly from the table.

• The person may turn blue and/or collapse.

Heimlich Remedy for Helping Someone Choking: If the person cannot speak, breathe, or cough, have someone call for emergency medical help *immediately,* while you—

Step 1: Stand behind the person and wrap your arms around his waist. Allow the person's head and upper body to hang forward.

Step 2: Make a fist with one hand. Grasp the fist with your other hand, placing the thumb side of the clenched fist against the person's abdomen—slightly above the navel and below the rib cage. *Caution:* Make sure your fist is *below* the rib cage or you can add to the person's problems by cracking his ribs.

Step 3: With a quick inward and upward thrust, press your fist into the person's abdomen. The lodged piece of food should pop right out. Repeat this action a second time if necessary.

Self-Help Heimlich: If you're alone, gulping down your food, and something gets lodged in your throat—

Step 1: Make a fist with one hand and place the thumb side against your abdomen.

Step 2: With the other hand, grab your fist and press your fist in and upward in sharp, thrusting moves.

Another method is to press your abdomen forcefully against the back of a chair or a railing, forcing air out of your lungs and the object to be expelled.

Self-Help for a Fish Bone That's Stuck: If you're at home alone, and a fish bone gets stuck in your throat, don't panic. (That's easy for me to say.) Rush to the kitchen, take a raw egg, and swallow it. Now's not the time to worry about cholesterol, especially if the egg slides the fish bone down.

Prevention: Cut meat into small, bite-sized pieces. Do not laugh or talk while you have food in your mouth. Booze dulls the reflexes, so if you're going to drink and eat, drink *after* you have eaten.

And remember: When you're eating at home alone, eat as though you're out on a first date with someone you're very attracted to. In other words, eat very slowly and thoroughly chew each mouthful before swallowing.

There's good cholesterol (HDL) and there's bad cholesterol (LDL).

Cholesterol is found only in foods that come from animals—that means meats, dairy products, eggs, and products made with these foods.

According to the standards set by the American Heart Association for the average person, the total daily fat intake should be no more than thirty percent of his/her total daily calories. Cholesterol intake should be a maximum of 100 milligrams per 1,000 calories consumed daily. If you eat 2,000 calories a day, you should limit your cholesterol intake to 200 milligrams. These formulas are sensible generalizations and should be modified to accommodate your individual condition.

There are books available that give you food breakdowns, including fat and cholesterol counts. We recommend that you get one to guide you in planning and sticking to a heart-healthy food regimen. Check the Health section in your local book store.

The American Heart Association categorizes fats and oils this way—

Not Recommended (saturated fats): Butter, Vegetable Shortening, Vegetable Fat, Bacon, Salt Pork, Suet, Lard, Chicken Fat, Meat Fat, Coconut Oil, Palm Kernel, and Palm Oil.

Recommended Oils (monounsaturated and polyunsaturated fats): Sunflower, Safflower, Corn, Soybean, Sesame Seed, Canola, and Olive Oil.

Ah, olive oil! It can actually *lower* the bad (LDL) cholesterol. That's not to say you're to guzzle it down. The key word is *moderation.* There's a big selection of olive oils on the market.

The one that's thought to have the most heart-protecting chemicals is extra virgin olive oil.

The following suggestions may help reduce your bad cholesterol and/or raise your good cholesterol.

TO LOWER BAD (LDL) CHOLESTEROL

• Eat brussels sprouts and other members of the cabbage family several times a week.

• Have raw garlic or garlic pills or liquid garlic extract daily.

• If you don't know from beans, it's time you start learning. A cup of beans a day can do a lot to lower cholesterol. And what a variety from which to choose: black beans, black-eyed peas, chickpeas, fava beans, kidney beans, lentils, lima beans, navy beans, pinto beans, split peas, white beans, and even canned baked beans.
Portions or dosages for the above should be determined by you and your health professional, depending on your cholesterol levels, size, and dietary needs.

• Eat raw carrots. Studies show that, in those who ate two and a half medium-sized raw carrots a day, blood cholesterol was lowered an average of eleven percent. The ingredient credited with the carrots' impressive results is calcium pectate.

• Eat turnips and/or rutabagas. Have them on a regular basis and they will ensure regularity as well as help your cholesterol.

• Eat broccoli . . . often. This tasty green-stalked beauty also has calcium pectate.

• Onions are rich in potassium and vitamin A as well as calcium pectate—all LDL fighters.

• A portion of oat bran or oatmeal is a great way to start the day. The beta-glucan in oats helps lower cholesterol.

• Eat soybeans and soybean products several times a week . . . at least. Don't make a face! There are delicious meatlike foods that can do you a world of good, especially when you consider that you'd be eating them in place of meat. Investigate.

Be adventurous. But remember, when you experiment with these "new-age" foods, you run the risk of getting healthier.

• Lecithin, derived from soybeans, comes in different forms—granules, capsules, and liquid. The granules have an interesting taste and texture. As we said before, be adventurous and experiment. The cholesterol you lower will be your own.

• Eating eggplant is said to rid the body of cholesterol before it can actually be absorbed by the body.

• Eat grapefruit as you would an orange. Peel it, separate it into sections, and enjoy. Come to think of it, eat oranges, too. The white skin covering the fruits and the membrane that separates the sections have pectin, the cholesterol-lowering ingredient.

• An apple or two a day . . . The peel has the pectin, so be sure to thoroughly clean it before eating it. (See HEALTHFUL AND HELPFUL HINTS for cleaning methods.)

TO RAISE GOOD (HDL) CHOLESTEROL

• Eat garlic—lots of it.

• Eat onions—lots of them.

• Take vitamin B-6 (100 mgs daily). It may raise the good cholesterol considerably. B-6 is extremely beneficial to smokers who have low HDLs.

Cholesterol-Free Vegetable Soup: To make a cholesterol-free soup, add extra water when cooking barley, millet, or brown rice and overcook it until it's a creamy consistency. Add steamed vegetables, take a spoon—and hearty appetite!

COLD SORES
(FEVER BLISTERS)

About eighty-five percent of all Americans get the dreaded cold sore. The unsightly sore is caused by the herpes simplex virus that bursts into bloom when resistance is low because of a cold, the flu, pregnancy, sunburn, or other metabolism-altering factors. It usually takes about two weeks to clear up. We have some suggestions that may speed up the healing process and prevent them from recurring—

COLD SORE REMEDIES

• Television producer Cyndi Antoniak, who got this unique cold sore remedy from her dermatologist, told us that there's a peculiar tingling feeling the second a cold sore is on its way. People who get cold sores will know exactly what she means. It's at that time that you take colorless nail polish and paint the area where the cold sore is about to emerge. The nail polish prevents the sore from blossoming. In fact, since Cyndi successfully used this remedy some time ago, she has not had a recurrence of cold sores. Incidentally, the polish peels off within a short time.

• Dry up the cold sore by applying ice to it. Place an ice cube in a white handkerchief and hold it on the sore for five minutes every hour. Okay, you want it on for a half-hour three times a day? Ten minutes ten times a day? Get the message? Keep the ice cube on as long as you can, as often as you can. Reports of this ice cube treatment say that the sores dry up in about two days.

• Apply yogurt or buttermilk to the sore to help dry it out.

• Zap a cold sore with vitamin E—400 IU. Puncture a capsule and squeeze out the oil and cover the sore with it. Do it three times a day. By the third application, you should no longer have pain. By the next day—the sixth application—the cold sore should be healed.

• Use aloe vera to help heal a cold sore. Break or cut a leaf, squeeze out the gel, and smear it on the sore. Do it three or four times a day, every day, until the sore is gone. If you don't have an aloe plant, you can buy aloe vera gel in a health food store.

• Put a half teaspoon of red wine in a saucer and leave it there for a few hours. Then scrape up the solidified remains of the wine and spread it on the cold sore. The pain should be gone in seconds; the cold sore will take a little longer to disappear.

Cure and/or Prevention: Daily doses of acidophilus can help heal and, better yet, prevent cold sores. You can take acidophilus in pill form (follow dosage on the label); and there's also acidophilus milk (two tablespoons daily). Yogurt with active culture and buttermilk also have the friendly bacteria thought to do battle with the herpes virus. For prevention, eat yogurt and drink buttermilk.

The herpes virus thrives on arginine, which is an amino acid. Stay away from these arginine-rich foods: chicken soup, chocolate, cola, nuts, gelatin, grain cereals, peas, and beer.

L-lysine is the amino acid that can inhibit the growth of the herpes virus. So include in your daily diet these foods that are rich in L-lysine: baked potatoes—lots of baked potatoes—brewer's yeast, and steamed flounder. Wouldn't you know, this list is not as appetizing as the no-no list.

Supplementing your diet with L-lysine tablets can be extremely effective in preventing cold sores or, at least, making them disappear quickly. Dosage ranges from 500 mgs to 4,500 mgs a day. Please check with a health professional to help you determine dosage.

Caution: If you're pregnant or are nursing, L-lysine may *not* be for you. Check with your obstetrician.

Further Prevention: Cold sores can be quite contagious. Do not hug, kiss, or shake hands with someone who has a cold sore. If *you* have the cold sore, be kind, but not affectionate.

And remember: The herpes virus thrives in bathrooms, where there's lots of moisture. Their perfect hangout is your tooth-brush. They can live there for days and then reinfect you. You may want to keep your toothbrush in a room that's less humid than the bathroom.

The second you think you're getting a cold sore, throw away the toothbrush you've been using and use a new one. This may prevent the cold sore from coming out. If you didn't catch it in time and the boo-boo blossoms, wait until it heals, then be sure to start using a new toothbrush again. It's important.

It's also important to keep the lip of your toothpaste tube away from your toothbrush so that you don't transmit the virus to the tube and infect your newest toothbrush.

𝒮 **Affirmation:** Repeat this affirmation at least fifteen times, first thing in the morning, last thing at night, and every time you look in the mirror—

I am strong. I am free. I radiate good health.

At any given time, an estimated five percent of all Americans have a cold. That's at least twelve million miserable people. It means the number of people with colds exceeds the number of people with all other ailments *combined.* It also means that there's a one-in-twenty chance you have a cold right now.

The common cold costs the country thirty million lost school and work days a year.

Fighting the *personal cold war* costs Americans approximately three billion dollars a year in doctor appointments and two billion dollars in remedies. Want to save two billion dollars? Consider some of our suggestions using ingredients you may already have in your home.

Universal Cure-Alls: Every nation has its own version of garlic and/or onion cold/flu remedies. Here are a few of the least complicated/most effective ones—

• Eat a raw or a roasted Spanish onion before bedtime . . . in the morning, no cold.

• Peel a clove of garlic, keep it in your cheek, and every so often, bite into it to release the potent juice. Change the clove every few hours. It is thought that the cold will be gone within twenty-four hours.

• Chop up a few cloves of garlic, wear them in a sac around your neck, and breathe in the vapors throughout the day.

• Take garlic/onion perles—follow the dosage on the label.

Drink a Guggle-Muggle. As we were growing up, we would see Bubbie, our grandmother, mix up a groan-provoking concoction whenever someone in the family had a cold. The dreaded drink was called a *Guggle-Muggle.* We thought it was a cute name that Bubbie made up.

One day, during Edward Koch's last term in office as mayor of the Big Apple, we had a bit of a surprise. The mayor had a cold and shared an ancient cure with all of New York—his family's recipe for a *guggle-muggle.*

It turns out that many Jewish families have their own guggle-muggle recipes . . . some more palatable than others. Our family's is the worst; Mr. Koch's is one of the best. As Ed Koch said, "It is not only medically superb, it is delicious!" And, with his permission, we share with you his for-adults-only guggle-muggle recipe.

Take the juice of one grapefruit, one lemon, and one orange, preferably a Temple orange—because of its taste and because of its name. Add one tablespoon of honey. Pour the mixture into a saucepan and bring it to a boil while stirring. Then add at least one ounce of your favorite liquor. (Brandy is Ed Koch's.)

As with most guggle-muggles, you drink it down and then get under the covers. Next morning, no cold.

An Anti-Everything for Colds and Flu: Bee propolis, the sticky sap of trees that's gathered and processed by bees, is an antihistamine, an antibiotic, an antivirus, antifungus, and also a decongestant. No kidding, it's amazing stuff! Bee propolis comes in tablets, capsules, and liquid form. Follow the dosage recommended on the label.

Note: If you have a suspected sensitivity to bee products, forget this and go on to other remedies.

Catching Colds: Tests were conducted between people with upper respiratory infections (colds) and people without colds. The tests consisted of kissing. The results suggested that the mouth and saliva are not the number one way colds are spread. Colds are most often transferred by nose-to-nose contact.

So, when you or your mate has a cold, kissing is fine . . . just keep your nose out of it!

At the Onset of a Cold: Peel and grate about a half-ounce of fresh ginger root and steep it in a cup of just-boiled water for ten minutes. Strain and drink a cup every couple of hours. If you like *hot and strong,* then add an eighth-teaspoon of cayenne pepper to the ginger tea. If you like *sweet,* add a tablespoon of raw honey to the ginger tea. If you like *tart,* add the juice of half a small lemon to the ginger tea.

To Prevent Dehydration: You know how they always say, "drink lots of liquids"? *They* are right. When you have a cold or the flu, and especially if you're running a fever, your body is throwing off water by means of evaporation, sweating, and breathing. We don't want to scare you by telling you how harmful dehydration can be, but we do want to impress upon you the need to keep replenishing that lost water. Keep drinking! The drinks above can help.

Chest Congestion: Boil a cup of white wine and carefully inhale the vapor to clear up chest congestion.

Or, after breakfast or lunch, add a half-teaspoon of Red Hot sauce to a glass of water and drink it. This remedy is so strong, you can almost feel congestion breaking up as the liquid goes down.

Sneezing: Do it! It's better to expel viruses and bacteria through sneezing than to stifle the sneezes, allowing the enemies to fester in your sinuses.

The best way to sneeze is with your mouth open and covered with a tissue.

Stuffed Nose: Upper body exercise can act as a natural nasal decongestant. Put on spirited music that arouses your passion and, pencil or chopstick in hand, conduct the band or orchestra that's playing the music. It's strenuous exercise, so you may not want to overdo your debut as guest conductor.

Runny Nose: Does your nose run? And do your feet smell? Then you're built upside down. But seriously . . . If you do have a runny nose, put three or four drops of Tabasco sauce in a glass of water and drink it down. Relief should be no more than five minutes away.

Color Therapy: Barbara Stabiner, clairvoyant and author, says to wear a red scarf around your neck to help speed the healing process.

Gem Therapy: To help clear up your cold, use a blue/green stone that has some clarity such as aquamarine, blue topaz, or blue tourmaline. (See RESOURCES for mail order gems.)

Aromatherapy: The minute you start feeling flu-ish, prepare a warm bath with a half dozen drops of cinnamon oil. Relax in the bath for fifteen minutes. Then, throughout the day, dab a little cinnamon oil on your temples.

When your head is feeling all stuffed up, fill the sink (or a bowl if you prefer) with hot water and put a couple of drops of cinnamon oil in it. Then place a towel over your head, your head over the sink, and inhale the cinnamon vapor for two or three minutes.

Visualization: "The River of Life," a visualization anyone can use to help get over a common cold, is by Dr. Gerald Epstein, from his book *Healing Visualizations* (Bantam Books, 1989):

> Once you're seated in a comfortable place, close
> your eyes. Breathe out three times to relax yourself.
> See your eyes becoming clear and very bright.
> Then see them turning inward, becoming two rivers
> flowing down from the sinuses into the nasal cavity
> and throat, their currents taking away all the waste
> products, soreness, and stuffiness. The rivers are
> flowing through your chest and abdomen, into your
> legs, and coming out as black or gray strands that
> you see being buried deep in the earth. See your
> breath coming out as black air and see your waste
> products emerging from below. Sense the rivers
> pulsating rhythmically through the body and see
> light coming from above, filling up the sinuses, nose,
> and throat, all the tissues becoming pink and
> healthy. When you sense both the rhythmic flow

and the light filling these cavities, breathe out and open your eyes.

Do this visualization exercise every three hours for three to five minutes each time, until the cold clears up.

𝒮 **Affirmation:** Repeat this affirmation five times. Each time you say it, think of how meaningful the words are and how they relate to you and your life.

My mind, my body, my work, and my relationships are clearly defined. I am in control. I am getting better and better. I am productive and I am loved.

Considering the selection of natural laxatives that are available, it seems to us that no one should have to resort to commercial products that can ultimately *cause* constipation.

Talk about causing constipation—you might want to limit your intake of the following foods that have been known to cause constipation: milk, cheese, ice cream, unripe bananas, heavily salted and spiced foods, chocolate, alcoholic beverages, and products made with white flour.

Our job is to provide nonchemical remedies that can help you become *regular;* your job is to try them—one at a time—using common sense and your doctor's approval. We suggest dosages. *More* is not always better. Take into account your size and system. Start with moderate amounts of whatever you want to try and experiment by gradually increasing the portion until you find what works for you.

NATURAL CONSTIPATION REMEDIES

• Have a few white or black mustard seeds daily. Swallow the seeds whole, without chewing them.

• First thing in the morning, eat a few figs or a very ripe banana. Eat another very ripe banana after dinner.

• Sprinkle two tablespoons of oat bran into food—soup, salad, or stew—each day.

• First thing in the morning, mix a tablespoon of cornmeal in a glass of water and drink it.

• Eat a ripe avocado—mix it with a little chopped onion, a teaspoon of lemon, and spices (curry or cumin) to taste.

• First thing in the morning, take one tablespoon of aloe vera juice (available at health food stores) and another tablespoon before bed.

• Peel and boil a sweet potato in water until it's soft. Eat it as your dinner dessert.

• First thing in the morning, drink a glass of grapefruit juice or fresh carrot juice.

• As an afternoon snack, eat a cup of cooked cabbage. It's a low-calorie, anti-cancer, fiber-filled food that can help conquer constipation.

• First thing in the morning, drink a glass of warm water with the juice of a lemon. Add some honey to make it delicious. Or forget the lemon and instead mix one tablespoon of honey in a glass of warm water and drink it first thing in the morning or right before going to bed.

• Put half a dozen cloves in a mug and add a half-cup of just-boiled water and let it steep overnight. Then, first thing in the morning, drink the clove water.

• For men only: Chew a tablespoon of raw pumpkin seeds daily. It's also wonderful for prostate health.

• Choose apples—baked and eaten for breakfast and before bed; eaten raw after every meal; or steamed with honey in place of the core and eaten after every meal. Be sure to wash off the pesticides (for instructions, see HEALTHFUL AND HELPFUL HINTS).

• First thing in the morning, drink a glass of vegetable juice. Use any palatable combination of these juices: tomato, cucumber, white radish, celery, fresh homemade sauerkraut, cabbage, beet, or carrot.

• Eat a salad, making sure you include a generous portion of sprouts—alfalfa, sunflower, radish, and/or lentil.

• Drink a couple of cups of bayberry tea (available at health food stores) every day.

• How can we suggest constipation remedies without mentioning the country's classic, all-natural laxative, the prune?

Overnight, soak four to six prunes in just-boiled water. In the morning eat the prunes and drink the water.

• Candy A-Go-Go: Process or finely chop ½ lb. of prunes, ½ lb. of raisins, ½ lb. of figs, and ¼ lb. of apricots, then combine them with ½ cup of unprocessed oat or wheat bran. Thoroughly mix the ingredients together. In an 8 inch square cake pan, evenly distribute the mixture. Cut into bite-sized squares, wrap each square in cellophane and keep the batch in the refrigerator. Eat 1 or 2 pieces daily.

• Finally, exercise on a regular basis. It can help make you regular. Rarely do joggers suffer from constipation.

Aromatherapy Bath: Put warm water in your bathtub along with a dozen drops of rosa gallica (available at most health food stores and herb shops). Relax in the tub for fifteen minutes or more. Do this three times a week.

Acupressure: Massage the area that's indented between your bottom lip and your chin. Just keep massaging and you should get results within fifteen minutes.

Compress: Take a white towel and carefully pour just-boiled water on it. When it's cool enough to touch, wring it out and put it on your stomach. To keep in the heat, place another towel over it. Now relax that way for a half hour. This can be done in conjunction with any of the above.

Colon Cleansing Regimen: You may want to help cleanse your colon on a regular basis by going on a fruit fast once a week or once a month—you set the schedule according to your needs and after checking with your health professional.

Be sure to include ripe pineapple, papaya, and/or mango. Also, in compliance with food combining, melons (cantaloupe, honeydew, watermelon, casaba, etc.) should be eaten by themselves to avoid gas buildup.

Or take advantage of psyllium, the beneficial fiber used in some commercial laxatives, without having the unnecessary commercial additives. Ask for powdered psyllium seed husks at health food stores and follow the directions on the label.

Note: You must have water with the psyllium and then have more water right after. Psyllium is mucilaginous; it absorbs water and gets clumpy. It can *cause* blockage if you don't wash it down with a generous supply of water.

Laugh Away the Problem: Really. Having a good laugh—a belly laugh—massages the intestines. It also relieves stress, a common cause of constipation. Rent a funny video; talk to a funny friend; or read the jokes in the "Well-Being" chapter of this book.

COUGHS

Coughing is your body's way of ridding itself of a substance somewhere along the respiratory tract. Most coughs are symptoms of respiratory ailments such as colds or the flu.

Here are remedies to help you deal with a cough. We suggest you go a step further and treat the cause of the cough as well.

At the Onset of a Cough: Prepare dill tea (available at health food stores) by adding one teaspoon of dill to a cup of just-boiled water. Let it steep for seven minutes, strain, if you need it sweetened, sweeten with honey, and drink three cups a day. All it may take to get rid of the cough are just those three cups for just that one day.

Cough Syrups: The classic folk remedies for coughs all seem to have honey as one of the main ingredients. These are no exception.

You can make cough syrup by putting a hole through the middle of a big onion or beet or turnip or rutabaga and filling it with honey, then roasting it.

Our favorite is to roast a big, juicy lemon until it splits open. Take a teaspoon of the lemon juice with a half teaspoon of raw honey every half hour until there's no more juice in the lemon. By then, the cough should be under control.

Cough Drops: This is the most complex recipe in the book. It was given to us by Ron Hamilton of Great American Natural Products and it's for those of you who are ready for the experience of making your own, natural, super-effective cough drops.

The ingredients are: a quarter-cup of dried horehound (available at health food and herb stores), two cups of water, two cups of honey, and one cup of blackstrap molasses.

Bring the water to a boil and add the horehound. Let it simmer for ten minutes. Strain and put the strained boiled horehound water in a large, heavy pot, along with the honey and blackstrap molasses. The mixture foams a lot, so be sure to use a large pot to avoid a messy range.

Cook the concoction for about an-hour-and-a-half and then start testing for readiness. When a drop of the mixture is dropped into cold water and becomes a hard ball, it is ready.

Carefully pour the mixture onto a very lightly buttered cookie sheet. Score it with a knife into cough-drop-size squares. When it cools, you will have very potent cough drops.

Decongestants: Eating spicy foods can help you cough up mucus and clear your lungs, sinuses, and nose. Get out the chili, horseradish, mustard, and garlic. Ah, garlic.

Prepare your own garlic cough syrup. Peel and mince six to eight cloves of garlic; put them in a jar with a cup of raw honey. Let this stand for two hours. Then, when your cough acts up, take a teaspoon of the syrup-and-garlic bits.

Garlic tea can also help clear up a cough. Add a quarter-teaspoon of garlic powder to a cup of just-boiled water. Or peel and mince three medium cloves of garlic and steep them in a cup of just-boiled water for ten minutes. Strain and drink the garlic tea—three or four cups a day—and add the minced garlic bits to soup or a salad.

Mucus and Cough Chaser: If you've reached the point where you feel your cough will never go away, fenugreek tea to the rescue! Start by drinking a cup of fenugreek (available at health food stores) every hour or two. After that first day, cut down to four cups each day.

Fenugreek is a powerful medicinal herb that can soften and wash away masses of mucus and clear up your cough in the process.

Bronchial Cough and Chest Congestion: A bay leaf poultice can work wonders to stop the cough and clear up the congestion. For fifteen minutes, steep twenty bay leaves in a covered cup of just-boiled water. Then separate the leaves from the liquid. Put the leaves in cheesecloth and moisten the cheesecloth by dipping it in the liquid. Place this wet bay leaf poultice on your bare chest and cover it with a towel. After an hour, reheat the liquid and re-dip the poultice and reapply it to your chest.

Aromatherapy for Bronchitis: Before bedtime, take a relaxing therapeutic bath. Scent the bath water with four drops of pine oil. If you find the familiar forest fragrance soothing, place a few drops of the oil on a cottonball and rub it on the back and undersides of wooden furniture, where the aroma will help alleviate the bronchitis throughout the day.

Dry, Hacking Cough: In cold weather, when windows stay closed and your home's heating system keeps the air dry, keep a pan of water on the radiator in your bedroom. It will humidify the air and help prevent a dry, hacking cough.

Cough with Phlegm: The owner of a Chinese restaurant shared this powerful, time-tested phlegm-ridding remedy with us. Grate a half-ounce of fresh ginger root into a cup of just-boiled water. While it's steeping, remove the meat from three walnuts. When the ginger tea has cooled down, drink the liquid and the grated ginger while eating the walnuts. (The ginger may be too strong for you to chew, so if you grate it finely, you can swallow it down without chewing.) Then go to bed and wake up in the morning phlegm-free and without the cough.

Choking Cough: This is the kind of cough where you are not actually choking on something—you're just coughing like that. All you have to do is raise your hands as high as you can and the choking cough will stop.

Morning Cough: If part of your morning routine consists of coughing, it's time to do something about it. Consider giving up mucus-making foods, especially dairy products . . . all dairy products. And instead of that cup of coffee, start the day with a cup of thyme tea. With thyme, within no time, you should have coughless mornings.

Postnasal Drip Cough: This is not a remedy for postnasal drip; it's a suggestion for quelling a postnasal drip cough and for getting some ZZZZZs. Sleep on your stomach! Now why didn't *you* think of that?

Nervous Cough: Drink an ounce of aloe vera juice (available at health food stores) first thing in the morning and right after dinner. It has been reported that the juice will help stop the nervous cough within a week.

Smoker's Cough: First, stop smoking! Did we lose you or are you still with us? Remove the peel, core, and seeds of six apples. Slice them in small pieces, add two cups of honey, and cook it on a low flame until it has a syrupy consistency. Let it cool, then put it in a jar and keep it refrigerated. Take two teaspoons of the honey-apple syrup between meals and whenever the cough acts up.

Now turn to the SMOKING section in this book, and fulfill your New Year's resolution.

♪ **Affirmation:** Repeat this affirmation at least twelve times, after each meal and at bedtime.

I am relaxed and surrounded by positive energy as my body heals itself.

❧Cuts and Wounds❧

If a cut or wound is bleeding profusely, put direct pressure on it with a sterile dressing and get professional medical help immediately.

If you have a minor cut, first rinse it with water, then dress it with any of these remedies to stop the bleeding:

- Crushed geranium plant leaves
- Goldenseal powder
- Papaya pulp
- Cayenne pepper
- Moist tea leaves
- Wet pouch tobacco
- Aloe vera plant leaf gel

When Help Isn't Close By: Our Massachusetts friend, Selwyn P. Miles, told us about a young lad who was chopping kindling on a farm. The axe slipped and caught him in the foot between his big and second toes. His dad scooped up a handful of honey from a crock and smeared it all over the boy's foot. The bleeding stopped instantly and complete healing followed in a short amount of time with little scarring. Selwyn emphasized that the remedy worked because of the enzymes in the raw honey.

SCARLESS HEALING:

• Carefully crack open a raw egg and remove the skin that's inside the shell. Put the wet side on the cut for a speedy healing without a scar.

• Once the wound closes, massage vitamin E oil on it daily, in the morning, at bedtime, and more often if possible.

• During her Mexican vacation, artist Barbara Wasserman was sent flying through a car's windshield. Her face was cut in several places. Considering all the stitches needed to close the cuts, Barbara was sure she'd be scarred for life. Luckily, while convalescing in Mexico, she had a local housekeeper who had been raised with folk remedies. The housekeeper took a big, beautiful abalone shell, put the juice of a lemon in it, and left it outside overnight in the moonlight. By morning, there was a paste formed by the lemon juice mixing with the pearlized part of the shell. The housekeeper gently applied the paste on the wounds. That night, she added more lemon juice on the shell and once again left it out overnight. This procedure was repeated daily—and every couple of weeks when the pearlized portion of the shell was used up, a new shell replaced it—until the wounds were completely healed and there was absolutely no trace of a facial scar.

When Barbara talked to us, she had just helped a friend who had had open-heart surgery. After a month of putting the abalone/lemon juice paste on his incision, just a faint hairline scar remained. "And that would completely disappear," Barbara said, "if my friend wasn't lazy about doing this for himself."

Barbara's friend put the paste on his chest in the morning. But Barbara, who had to have it on her face, put it on at bedtime. That way she didn't have to wash it off to go out. Barbara also told us that you don't have to put the shell outside under the moon. A dark closet overnight is adequate.

We experimented with shells and juice and found that it may take *two* nights for the juice to eat through the top layer of shell enough to form a usable paste.

If you have a *fresh* scar-producing incision and want to try this remedy, we urge you to check with your health professional and take every precaution against infection.

Depression is known as the common cold of mental illness. According to the National Institute of Mental Health's Office of Scientific Information, depression affects over ten million adults each year. Now that's depressing.

Depression doesn't discriminate. It affects the rich and famous as well as the poor and unknown. In 1841, when Abraham Lincoln was the floor leader of the Whig party, he was quoted as saying, "If what I feel were equally distributed to the whole human family, there would not be one cheerful face on earth." Yes, Mr. Lincoln was going through a depression. He eventually conquered it and went on to become the sixteenth president of the United States.

Another case in point—Winston Churchill. Sir Winston took up painting to help him get through his bouts of depression.

If an artist's palette isn't palatable to you, you might want to consider the following suggestions—

Myrrh, one of the presents given to the Christ child by the three kings, is said to chase the blues away. Put a half teaspoon of powdered myrrh (available at health food stores) in a cup of just-boiled water. Let it cool and drink it twice a day.

Many psychic practitioners believe that burning myrrh incense chases away negative energy.

Okay, everyone on your feet, two, three, four. Yes, exercise can take the place of antidepressant drugs and have the same effect on the chemicals of your brain that give you a feeling of well-being . . . and without any of the drugs' side effects other than getting into great shape.

Take a good, brisk walk every day, setting your own personal best records. Rent or buy an exercise video tape—make sure it's at your own workout level—and start working out. Join a gym or health club and make a commitment to yourself to work out on a daily basis. Exercise can almost immediately make you feel better about yourself and about life in general.

Vitamin B-6 is the answer for some people who are in a depressed state. Magnesium is needed for the most effective absorption of vitamin B-6. Magnesium along with calcium can calm the nervous system and help relieve depression. Are you still with me? To simplify things, if you're interested in this remedy, the dosage is 100 mgs of B-6, 100 mgs of magnesium, and 200 mgs of calcium—all twice a day.

Caution: Check with your doctor before you try this remedy. Have him/her approve the dosages for you.

Warning: Do not take more than 250 mgs of vitamin B-6 a day. It can be toxic.

A word to women on the Pill: The estrogen in the Pill can stop the absorption of vitamin B-6, along with several other vitamins and minerals. That absorption may be the cause of your depression. You might want to consider another means of birth control. Check with your doctor to know what's available to you.

Get out of a mild depression by getting out and doing some gardening. Indoor gardening is good, too. According to the National Horticultural Therapy Association, growing plants can give you a new appreciation for life and a chance to *bury* your unhappiness. Join Plant Parenthood now!

After a Loss: Native Americans used borage to help comfort the bereaved "when the heart weeps with sorrow." Prepare tea by steeping one heaping teaspoon of borage (available at health food stores) in a cup of just-boiled water for ten minutes, then strain and drink. Three cups of this tea (it has a cucumber taste) can do a lot to ease emotional pain and grief.

After a Loss or Any Other Major Trauma: Get into therapy by going into a stationery store and buying a special pad or book to use as an emotional diary. At least once a day, write down your innermost feelings. Don't censor yourself; let it all out on paper. The purging of your thoughts and emotions can help speed the healing process, assist in the management of your grief, and help prevent you from suppressing all that you need to release. When you've completed the process and are a lot better, you may want to continue with the diary.

Are You a SAD-ist?: If, during the dark months of winter, you consistently experience one or more of these symptoms—depression, moodiness, lethargy, problems sleeping, and a bigger-than-usual appetite along with a craving for carbohydrates—you may be one of the five percent of Americans with Seasonal Affective Disorder (SAD).

Lack of exposure to sunlight seems to be the cause. For mild cases, the recommended treatment is that you spend more time outdoors in winter. (Sitting indoors, near a window, doesn't do it.) For severe cases, SAD sufferers need phototherapy. That means either visits to a light room at a clinic or lab, or investing in banks of full-spectrum lights that can be used in your home.

Visualization: Dr. Gerald Epstein's visualization, "Blowing Away the Dark Clouds," is for people who have a general feeling of blueness. This process can rid you of that feeling. Sit on a comfortable, hard-back chair, relax, and take up to a minute for this process.

Close your eyes and see dark clouds above you. As you stand under these clouds, see yourself blowing them away to the left by blowing out three breaths (in imagery, *not* physically). Then look up in the sky to the upper right and watch the sun enter the sky above you. When finished, know that the blues have gone.

Slowly count from one to three. Open your eyes, stretch, and feel refreshed and happier.

Gem Therapy: Clairvoyant and author Barbara Stabiner says that the sapphire contributes to mental clarity, aids in perception and discernment, is used for protection, and acts as an anti-depressant.

♫ **Affirmation:** Repeat this Jose Silva affirmation (based on French psychotherapist Émile Cové's words) first thing in the morning, throughout the day—the second you catch yourself thinking a negative thought—and last thing at night. Say it at least ten times—

Every day in every way I'm getting better, better, and better.

REFERRAL

For depression information and referrals to other organizations, call or write to:

National Mental Health Association
1021 Prince Street
Alexandria, VA 22314-2971
800/969-NMHA

According to the Centers for Disease Control, over fourteen million Americans have diabetes; at least half don't know it.

If there's a family history of diabetes and/or you have *any* of the symptoms, have your health care provider test you for it.

The symptoms are: frequent urination, unquenchable thirst, increased appetite, weight loss, and in some cases, itching of the skin.

When you have diabetes, your pancreas doesn't produce the amount of insulin needed to metabolize sugar. When you have diabetes, you no longer have the luxury of letting your body go on automatic. You have to consciously take control in three ways—diet, exercise, and diligent monitoring under the supervision of your health care provider.

The diabetic diet is a sensible one. We've heard from people who were devastated when they found out they had diabetes. They changed their eating habits to conform with a diabetic diet and feel better, look better, and are healthier now than they've been in years.

An exercise program is important because it helps burn up sugar, and may prevent complications that can be caused by the condition, for instance, high blood pressure or poor circulation.

For more information, see Referral for a contact. For some self-help tips, read on—

Adult-Onset Diabetes Prevention: An adequate daily amount of the trace mineral chromium can prevent millions of people from developing adult-onset diabetes, according to Dr. Richard A. Anderson of the U.S. Department of Agriculture.

Dr. Anderson says that people with a minor glucose intolerance—one-fourth of all Americans—are the ones most likely to develop diabetes. Chromium stimulates insulin to perform better in an impressive eighty-five percent of those people, helping prevent adult-onset diabetes.

Just fifty micrograms of chromium a day could make the difference. Take a multivitamin/mineral supplement and/or eat foods rich in chromium—brewer's yeast, clams, wheat bran and other whole grain cereals, fruits, and vegetables . . . especially broccoli.

We've all heard talk of how behavior changes when there's a full moon. Researchers are saying that there is something to it; you can be "moonstruck." If you have diabetes, check your calendar and be *extra* careful and conscientious with your diet and your medication when there's a full moon.

To better control a diabetic condition with diet, keep a food and drink diary and, *with the supervision of a health professional,* monitor your intake and the outcome.

You should know about the following foods and herbs that are known to help lower blood sugar levels and boost the manufacturing of insulin:

• Legumes—black beans, black-eyed peas, fava beans, lentils, and chickpeas to name a few of the high-fiber, blood-sugar-lowering and "bad"-cholesterol-lowering edibles.

• Try bulgur in place of rice.

• Jerusalem artichokes—a.k.a. sunchokes—eat two or three a day, raw, in place of a fruit, or in salads.

• Yarrow tea—two to four cups a day.

• Dandelion—said to be the best overall herb for diabetics. Eat fresh dandelion greens and, on the days you're not drinking yarrow tea, drink a few cups of tea made from dried dandelion leaves or roots (available at health food stores).

• Blueberry leaf tea—when you're not drinking the yarrow or dandelion teas, drink tea made from blueberry leaves (available at health food stores). It contains myrtillin, an ingredient that helps reduce blood sugar levels.

REFERRAL

For more information, call or write to:

American Diabetes Association
1660 Duke Street
Alexandria, VA 22314
800/ADA-DISC (Diabetes Information Service Center)

DIARRHEA

Believe it or not, an occasional bout of diarrhea can be a good thing. Diarrhea is your body's way of cleansing itself when it obviously needs to. For that reason, some health practitioners feel that you should wait six to eight hours before doing anything to stop the condition. (That's easy for them to say.)

Diarrhea can be caused by mild food poisoning, lactose intolerance (an allergic reaction to milk), a minor bacterial infection, fatigue, stress, overeating, or eating while upset or very nervous.

Whatever the cause of the condition, it causes depletion and dehydration. During a bout of diarrhea, you lose fluid that contains electrolytes—valuable minerals including potassium, chloride, sodium, magnesium, and calcium. It's a good idea to buy one of the sports beverages containing electrolytes that are now available at health food stores, to replace those lost minerals and restore your nutrient balance quickly. Also, be sure to drink lots of water throughout the diarrhea and after, too (mineral water seems best). Eat "binding" foods rich in those lost nutrients: whole grains like brown rice and barley, bulgur, potatoes with the skin, ripe bananas, and dark green leafy vegetables, lightly cooked.

Give your system a chance to get back to itself by not taxing it with fatty, oily foods, sugar and sugar products, white flour products, milk and milk products, and chocolate.

Now that you have an understanding of the problem, here is a selection of remedies to help solve it.

Caution: If you still have diarrhea after two full days of remedy-taking, check with your health professional to make sure it isn't a symptom of something else.

DIARRHEA REMEDIES

• To destroy the harmful bacteria that's causing the condition, drink a tablespoon of apple cider vinegar in a glass of water before each meal.

• Place an ice pack in the middle of the back and another one on the lower back—ten minutes on and ten minutes off, ten minutes on, etc., as long as these back packs seem to make you feel better.

• Drink one heaping teaspoon of cornstarch in a glass of water. If this doesn't help in two to three hours, then try another remedy.

• The classic folk remedy for diarrhea, dating back to biblical times, is blackberry—juice, wine, jam, brandy—just about any form of it. Recommended dosage every four hours: six ounces of blackberry juice; two ounces of blackberry wine; one heaping teaspoon of blackberry jam; or two tablespoons of blackberry brandy.

• Mix a rounded tablespoon of carob powder (available at health food stores) in a glass of warm water and drink it before each meal.

• Apples are wonderful for stopping diarrhea. Clean an apple according to the instructions in the HEALTHFUL AND HELPFUL HINTS chapter. Then grate the apple and let it stand until it turns brown. In other words, you're letting the pectin in the fruit oxidize, duplicating the basic ingredient in some popular over-the-counter diarrhea drugs. Once the grated apple turns brown, eat it. You might want to mix in some carob powder (see remedy above).

• Cinnamon is also helpful in correcting this condition. Sprinkle a quarter of a teaspoon of cinnamon powder on a grated apple.

Acupressure: Lie down, relax, and take the heel of your palm and place it on your navel. Press in and, in a circular motion, massage the area for a few minutes. It can help.

Traveler's Diarrhea Prevention: In foreign countries, drink carbonated bottled water instead of plain bottled water. Carbonation helps kill infection-causing microbes that can cause diarrhea or worse.

Traveler's Diarrhea: Worldwide health agencies and United States health services recommend this remedy when you're traveling out of the country and you get diarrhea. You need two glasses: In one glass pour eight ounces of distilled water and add a quarter teaspoon of baking soda; in the other glass pour eight ounces of orange juice, or any fruit juice and add a half-teaspoon of honey and a pinch of salt. Drink a mouthful from one glass, then from the other. Keep going back and forth until you finish the contents of both glasses and know relief is on its way.

𝒮 **Affirmation:** Repeat this at least ten times, every time you go to the bathroom and right before you make a phone call—

I accept myself for the perfect person I am. My mind and body are in harmony with the universe.

Voltaire described ears as "the roads to the heart." Moses Ibn Ezra referred to ears as "the gates to the mind." And Abraham Coles called them "bony labyrinthean caves." Roads, gates, or caves, here are suggestions for their well-being, so lend us your ears.

When the heat's on, the earache starts to go away. We have an unusual variety of remedies that supply heat:

• Place a white washcloth in a microwaveable container of water and zap it in the microwave for forty-five seconds. Then place the cloth on the ear.

• Sit in a car that has the sun shining in. Position your ear so that you feel the warm rays of the sun on it. As soon as the earache is gone, you, too, can take off.

• Set your hair dryer on warm, hold it a foot and a half from you, and direct the air into your ear.

• In a frying pan, warm a cup of kosher (coarse) salt, then funnel it into a white sock and cover your ear with it.

• If you get an earache as you're making breakfast, or while you're at the International House of Pancakes, put a pancake on your ear . . . without the butter and syrup.

Urine Cure: This age-old remedy doesn't require a trip to the store, is easy to do, and the price is right. Collect an ounce of your urine, and with a medicine dropper, put a few drops in your ear. Gently plug the ear with a cotton ball. Word has it that Elvis Presley's mother, who was into folk remedies, would have

Elvis give her a specimen that she would then use as eardrops for him whenever he had an earache.

Garlic Cure: Puncture a garlic perle and squeeze out the contents into your ear. Gently plug the ear with a cotton ball. It can help relieve the pain real fast.

Vodka Cure: With a medicine dropper, put three or four drops of room temperature vodka in the ear canal. We were told it takes the pain away in five minutes.

Reflexology: If your earache is due to being out in cold, windy weather, vigorously massage the tip of your fourth toe, the one next to the pinky, for instant relief.

If the earache has something to do with sinus congestion, massage the roof of your mouth.

Ear Problem Prone: If your ears are your Achilles heel, then you're built awfully funny. But seriously . . . If you seem to have ear infections more often than once in a blue moon, the irritants in cigarette smoke may be a contributing factor. *Do not smoke!* Don't even hang around people who are smoking. Ya hear?

Swimmer's Ear Prevention: If you keep getting swimmer's ear, try an ounce of prevention . . . make that a few drops of prevention. Right before you go swimming, put a few drops of either jojoba oil (available at health food stores) or mineral oil in each ear. That should put an end to your recurring swimmer's ear. Or: Within an hour of getting out of the water, blow up a balloon 3 or 4 times, or if you're having a beach party, blow up 3 or 4 balloons. The balloon-blowing process will prevent the infection that causes swimmer's ear.

Swimmer's Ear: If you did not follow the preventive measures above and you have swimmer's ear, you might want to try this:

Tip your head to the side and, using a medicine dropper, fill the ear with a solution of equal amounts of white vinegar and alcohol. Grab hold of your lobe and rotate it in a circular motion to make sure the liquid reaches the bottom of the ear canal. Then, tip your head the other way, allowing the liquid to empty out.

A Bug in Your Ear: It can happen . . . fortunately, not very often. If it happens in the dark, shine a flashlight in your ear. The insect should move or fly to the light. If it happens in daylight, a piece of fruit—an apple or peach—should be held at the ear. It should whet the insect's appetite, especially if it's a fruit fly.

Other Foreign Objects: On that extremely rare occasion when you get a little object in your ear, here's something to try before seeking professional help. Put two or three drops of olive oil in the ear, then gently smell black pepper—enough to make you sneeze. As you're about to sneeze, close your mouth and your nostrils. That way, the sneeze might cause the ear to pop out the object. (How did you get something in your ear to begin with?!)

Itchy Ears: Stop the itching by putting your head down with the itchy ear up. With a medicine dropper, fill the ear with apple cider vinegar. Leave it there for half a minute, then tilt your head to the other side and let the vinegar empty out.

Hearing Loss Prevention: According to a recent study, a low-cholesterol eating plan helps prevent hearing loss. Researchers found that the flow of blood through the small arteries in the ear is limited by cholesterol, resulting in loss of hearing. After thousands of people were monitored, the study concluded that hearing improved on a low-fat diet; on a fatty foods diet, hearing got worse.

Ringing in the Ears (Tinnitus): Over thirty million Americans have chronic tinnitus. Since it's actually a symptom rather than an ailment, the thing to do is to find out what is causing the symptom—medication, specifically salycilates (the active ingredient in aspirin), or mental trauma, or reaction to a loud noise.

If the cause is medication, once you stop taking it, the ringing usually stops. If you're still searching for the cause, drink fenugreek seed tea. Prepare the tea by adding a teaspoon of fenugreek seeds (available at health food stores and herb shops) to a cup of just-boiled water and let it steep for twenty minutes. Strain and drink a cup in the morning, another in the afternoon, and again at bedtime. Give it a couple of weeks to see results— uh, to *hear* results.

Gingko capsules (available at health food stores) can also help stop the ringing. Take forty mgs three times a day, for at least two weeks.

Gem Therapy for Inner Ear Problems: According to Barbara Stabiner, clairvoyant and author, amber is the stone for inner ear problems. Wear a piece of amber around your neck, tape it to your ear, or hold it in your hand.

Ears and Air Travel: In a plane, before you adjust to the difference in air pressure, your ears can be greatly affected . . . it can be a real pain in the ascent, as well as the descent, of course.

The act of swallowing opens the eustachian tube, which allows the pressure to equalize. Many passengers simply chew gum, suck candy, or yawn during the plane's takeoff and landing to feel comfortable.

For those of you who need something more, try the procedure recommended by the American Council of Otolaryngology. As soon as the plane takes off, hold both nostrils closed with your thumb and index finger, then take a mouthful of air. Using your cheek and throat muscles, force air into the back of your nose, as though you were trying to blow your fingers off your nostrils. While you're doing that, you should hear a pop in your ears. That means that equalization has been accomplished.

♪ **Affirmation:** Repeat this affirmation fifteen times, starting first thing in the morning, after each meal, and throughout the day, whenever you think to do it. The more often, the better.
I hear healing words of wisdom and love. I listen and learn.

REFERRAL

For the only completely hypoallergenic earring with a
lifetime guarantee against discomfort, write, fax, or call
for a catalog:

Roman Research, Inc.
33 Riverside Drive
Pembroke, MA 02359
Fax: 617/826-5550
800/225-8652

Eyes

Eyes—the windows of the soul, the heart's letter, those silent tongues of love, the spectacles of the brain, the organs through which intelligence shines, the contractors of cataracts, the blinkers that get bloodshot, the sources of sties . . .

Here are some suggestions that may help you . . . in the twinkle of an eye.

Note: If symptoms persist, be sure to consult with an eye doctor.

Sties: The classic sty remedy is to take a gold wedding ring and rub the blossoming sty with it. Some people believe it works better if you rub the ring on cloth until it's warm and then rub the sty with it.

This technique is given in our first folk remedy book, and it's the one we've gotten the most mail on. Letters usually start with, "We thought you were crazy but . . ." and then the writers go on to tell of their instant relief with the ring and the disappearance of their sty.

If you prefer, carefully dab a little aloe vera gel on the sty throughout the day—four or five times.

Or, collect your first urine of the day and dab a drop of it on your sty. Oh, grow up! After you do it in the privacy of your bathroom and the sty goes away, you may even share this remedy with friends.

Bloodshot Eyes and Eyestrain: What better name than eyebright for an herb that can soothe sore eyes, alleviate eyestrain, and clear up bloodshot eyes?

Mix one ounce of eyebright—the whole dried herb—into a pint of just-boiled water. Let it steep for ten minutes, then strain through a superfine strainer or through unbleached muslin. Drink a cup of the tea. Use the other cup of tepid tea for dipping cotton pads and place them on your closed eyes. Stay that way for fifteen minutes.

Alternatively, take two tablespoons of ginger powder and add enough water to make a runny paste. Smear it on the soles of your feet, put socks on top, and sleep that way. (To protect your linens, you may want to put plastic on the sheet under your feet.) In the morning, your eyes should look and feel fine.

You might also try making a poultice out of grated apple or grated potato. Lie down and put the poultice over your eyes for twenty minutes. The poultice will repair, nourish, and strengthen the eyes; relaxing for twenty minutes will take care of the rest of you.

Computer Eyestrain Prevention: The National Institute of Occupational Safety and Health recommends that you take a fifteen-minute break every hour when working at a computer's video display terminal. Also, position the screen at eye level about twenty-two to twenty-six inches away. The two tips can prevent or at least minimize eyestrain. (See more of the Institute's recommendations for computer users in HEALTHFUL AND HELPFUL HINTS.)

Gem Therapy for Eyestrain: Azurite, a beautiful blue stone, is recommended for eyestrain. It's said to be beneficial for sight as well as for insight. It's used to improve vision and visionary powers. To use azurite, put a stone on the inner corner of each eye—lids closed, of course. Stay that way for twenty minutes.

Gem Therapy for Bloodshot Eyes: The bloodstone (heliotrope), a dark green stone with blood red or orange oxide spots, is recommended for bloodshot eyes. Put a stone on the inner corner of each eye—lids closed, of course. Stay that way for twenty minutes.

Blurred Vision: Alfalfa tablets (available at health food stores) are said to help clear up one's vision. Completely dissolve one alfalfa tablet in a cup of just-boiled water. Let it cool, strain it through unbleached muslin, and bottle it. Put one drop of the solution in each eye every morning. Also add fresh alfalfa sprouts to your diet. They are a truly rejuvenating food.

Men, if you wear a tie that's too tight, it can actually inhibit the flow of blood to the brain and, in turn, blur your vision. You'll know your collar is too tight when you can't slip your finger between your neck and the shirt collar.

Cinders: When you have a cinder or something similar in your eye and you just can't get it out, take a flax seed and put it in that troubled eye. Bandage the eye and sleep that way overnight. In the morning, when you take off the bandage, the flax seed will have dislodged the cinder and both will fall out.

If a flax seed is too uncomfortable in your eye, use a chia seed. It's smaller. Wet the seed with your own saliva before putting it in your eye. When the seed is wet, it becomes mucilaginous. That means it's like a magnet, attracting things to itself, like the cinder. Once you've given it enough time to fulfill its mission, gently move it to the corner of the inner eye with a tissue and remove it. Hey, you can be your own chia pet.

"Gucky" Eyes: Separate the yolk from the white of a raw egg. Take cotton pads, dip them in the egg white, and place the pads on your eyes. Bind them in place and sleep that way. In the morning, your eyes should be clear.

Contact Lens Wearers' Dry Eyes: Vitamin B-6 (100 mgs twice a day) has been known to completely eliminate the discomfort of dry eyes within no time.

Warning: Do not take more than 250 mgs of vitamin B-6 a day. It can be toxic.

Contact Lens General Tip: Do not use hair spray while you're wearing contact lenses. The spray can coat the lenses with a hard-to-remove film.

Onset of a Cataract: Take the leaves of a jade plant. They're available at nurseries and florists and are inexpensive. Put the leaves in a pan with a little water on a medium fire for a couple of minutes until the leaves are hot. Once they're cool, squeeze out the juice. Put a couple of drops of that juice in the eye every morning for three weeks. It has been known to rid the eye of the cataract forever.

Note: *Be sure to check with your eye doctor before doing this.*

Eyesight Strengthener: Many Asian herbalists believe that chewing a very small piece of ginger after each meal can help improve one's eyesight. It will also help with digestion and gas.

Improve Night Vision: If you have a problem seeing at night, bilberry and zinc can help improve your vision. Both are available at health food stores. Take 80 mgs of bilberry twice a day. Men should also take 50 mgs of zinc daily; women should take 25 mgs of zinc daily.

Caution: Prolonged use of zinc can cause a copper deficiency. This remedy should be taken for a limited time only. If it's going to help, chances are you will *see* results within a month.

♪ **Affirmation:** For any kind of eye problem, repeat this affirmation twelve times, starting first thing in the morning, every time you see your favorite color, and last thing at night.

While you're at it, if it's logistically practical, rub your hands together until you feel the warmth you've created. Then cup your hands over your eyes, keeping them there as you say the affirmation a dozen times—

I see everything in my life happening for my greatest good and I'm finding joy in each day.

REFERRAL

Thanks to the National Eye Care Project, financially disadvantaged senior citizens over age sixty-five, can get medical and surgical eye care at no out-of-pocket cost. For more information call: 800/222-EYES

FATIGUE

We hear complaints from lots of people that they're always tired . . . that they lack energy . . . that they have no get-up-and-go. For the most part, their days start early in the morning and end late at night, with all kinds of responsibilities, pressures, obligations, and tension in between. For you people who fit the description above, it may be time to rethink the life you've created for yourself and make some changes.

While you're taking a good, close look at your lifestyle, we have some fatigue fighters in the form of instant revivers, energy boosters, and drowsiness-enders.

Instant Reviver: When you're sitting at a meeting and you're afraid you're going to nod off when you need to be alert and responsive, press your elbows against your sides, or press your knees together, exerting a lot of pressure for just a few seconds. Your blood circulation will be increased, making you feel more with it.

The Amazing Kreskin's Amazing Touch of Energy: If you've ever seen the Amazing Kreskin, world's foremost mentalist, perform—and who hasn't?—you know the tremendous level of energy there. The man is a dynamo! When we asked Kreskin the secret of his stamina, he generously shared his recipe with us—

Combine six ounces of unsweetened cranberry juice and two ounces of orange juice. Top it off with a slice of fresh lime, add ice, stir, and drink.

Kreskin consumes about a quart of his energy drink daily.

That seems a little excessive for the average person who doesn't have Kreskin's hectic show biz schedule. One eight-ounce drink a day sounds like a good picker-upper.

An Ounce of Prevention: Many is the afternoon I've almost dozed off over my computer keyboard, until I discovered the secret of staying awake. Eat a light lunch. Hamburger and fries?—No! Salad?—Yes! When weather permits, a short walk after lunch will go a long way in helping keep you wide-awake and alert the rest of the day.

Breathing "Right": In keeping with many who believe that positive energy is inhaled through the right nostril, put a piece of cotton in your left nostril and breathe through your right nostril for an hour. If you can be by yourself in a quiet space for that hour, so much the better in terms of your revitalization.

Energy Boosters: Instead of a *coffee* break, eat a handful of raw, unsalted sunflower seeds (available at health food stores). This high-powered protein nosh will do wonders for your energy level throughout the day.

Or try bee pollen: The more research we do on bee pollen, the more convinced we are that it's a miracle food. It can give you energy and stamina. In fact, many athletes are now using pollen in place of steroids or other harmful supplements.

Warning: Some people are allergic to bee pollen. Start very slowly—with a couple of granules the first day or two; then if you have no allergic reaction, work your way up gradually until you take one teaspoon or more a day.

You can get bee pollen at your local health food store, or check RESOURCES for our mail order recommendations.

Winter Fatigue: If you notice that you feel particularly tired *only* during the winter months, it may be due to Seasonal Affective Disorder (SAD). See DEPRESSION for an explanation and solution.

Chronic Fatigue: Many believe that chronic tiredness may be caused by vitamin deficiencies due to an unbalanced diet. Eat foods rich in the B-complex vitamins—whole grain cereal, brewer's yeast, and yogurt—and supplement your diet with a B-complex vitamin.

Eat foods rich in vitamin C—citrus fruits, leafy green vegetables, cabbage—and supplement your diet with 500 to 1,000 mgs of vitamin C spaced out through the day.

Also, eat foods rich in magnesium—whole grains, beans, dark green vegetables, soy products, and nuts.

Visualization for Drowsiness: Sit back, close your eyes, and let all the air out of your lungs. Imagine a bright blue-white energizing light entering and filling your entire body as you inhale slowly through your nostrils. Open your eyes and feel refreshed.

Aromatherapy for Drowsiness: Put a drop of allspice or cinnamon oil on the inside of your wrist and take a whiff every time your eyelids start feeling heavy.

If you have a real bad case of the drowsies, puncture a garlic perle and take a few deep whiffs. That ought to wake you up.

If you're at home and need to get your second wind for the evening, add six drops of lemon, peppermint, or thyme oil to your bath water. Relax in the bath for fifteen minutes.

Note: *If there's any chance you'll fall asleep in the tub, forget this remedy; try another.*

♪ **Affirmation:** Repeat this affirmation a dozen times, the second you feel yourself dragging—

I'm happy, healthy, awake, inspired, and raring to go.

Putting on spirited music and repeating the affirmation while listening to the music is even more effective.

According to Charles S. Smith in *Ten Steps to Comfort,* a person weighing 135 pounds takes close to 19,000 steps during an average day, absorbing a cumulative pressure of more than 2.5 million pounds. No wonder we have problems with our feet. Here are some solutions:

Athlete's Foot: Athlete's foot is a fungal infection whose siblings are jock itch and ringworm. What a family!

The fungus thrives in dark, warm, moist places—your shoes in the case of athlete's foot.

It takes at least a full day for shoes to dry thoroughly after being worn. No wonder—the average pair of feet give off a half-pint of perspiration daily. And so, don't wear the same pair of shoes two days in a row.

Avoid reinfecting your feet—by wiping out your shoes with vinegar. To be on the safe side, you might also rinse your socks with white vinegar, as well as the bathtub, shower, and bathroom floor.

Here are some remedies to consider:

• Before bedtime, soak the infected foot in apple cider vinegar for ten minutes. It will sting, but only for a few seconds. Then, moisten gauze with the cider vinegar and put it on the infection, binding it in place with a white handkerchief or Ace bandage and covering it with a sock. Keep it that way overnight and repeat the process the following morning, if possible. If not, wear clean hose during the day and repeat the process every evening until the infection clears up. It should take about two weeks.

• Apply aloe vera to the foot once in the A.M. and again in the P.M. You can buy aloe gel or juice in health food stores, or if you have an aloe plant, squeeze out the natural gel from a cut leaf.

We've been told that consistent applications of aloe have cleared up cases of chronic athlete's foot.

• Set aside an hour a day to dip your fungal foot in pineapple juice. When the timer goes off, thoroughly dry the foot and spread baking soda on the affected area.

• The external use of urine for medicinal purposes goes back hundreds of years. Did I just lose you, or are you still with me?

When our body is under attack, it fights back by manufacturing antibodies and sending them to do battle. These antibodies can be found in our urine. We can take advantage of that fact by using the urine externally to clear up athlete's foot.

Collect a specimen in a bowl and dip your foot in it for ten minutes. Do it in the morning and in the evening. Yes, you can wash your foot with water afterward.

It costs less than the (above) pineapple juice and it *almost* looks the same.

Acupressure for Athlete's Foot: Yes, there's an acupressure point that can help clear up this condition. The point is between the little piggy that had no roast beef and the one that went all the way home. In case you're not into nursery rhymes, the acupressure point is where the fourth toe and the little toe meet on the front of your foot. First thing in the morning, press that spot for ten seconds, then another ten seconds, and a third ten seconds. At night, press that spot again for ten seconds, three times in a row. It's hard to believe that it could help. It can, and as long as it won't *hurt* the condition, it's worth a try—along with one of the other remedies above.

Toenail Fungus: Puncture a vitamin E capsule (400 IU) and squeeze out the oil onto the nail. Keep it uncovered as much as possible and reapply the oil often. Soak infected toenails for 15 minutes a day in a combination of 1 part white vinegar to 2 parts water.

Or, see the "urine" remedy above.

Fungus Prevention: Raw garlic is a powerful fungus fighter. Eat one or two cloves a day and you may never have athlete's foot or toenail fungus.

Ingrown Toenail: At bedtime, put a slim wedge of lemon on the problem toenail, keeping it in place with a Band-Aid and covering it with a sock. Sleep that way, and by morning the lemon should have softened the nail enough to ease it away from the skin so you can trim it.

Cut the nail straight across, not down at the sides, and not shorter than the toe.

Tired, Aching Feet: Put up a pot of barley or millet—two cups of the grain to eight cups of water. As soon as it's thick-soup consistency, take it off the stove. When it's cool enough to handle, divide the mush into plastic shoeboxes, or a pan or basin large enough for your feet, and put your feet in.

Let the warm mush embrace your barking dogs for at least a half hour, then rinse with cold water and wipe dry with a rough towel.

You and your feet should feel rejuvenated.

Incidentally, you can reheat the barley or millet and use it again the next day and the next.

Hot, **Tired, Aching Feet:** Take a basin that's large enough for both of your feet and fill it with one layer of ice cubes—the melonball kind are the best for this. If you don't have a large enough basin, use a plastic shoebox and do one foot at a time. Sit down and rub your feet over the ice cubes. Stop when this massage has your feet feeling completely revitalized, or the ice melts—whichever comes first. Dry your feet with a rough towel. Ready for the marathon?

Shooting, Spasmodic Foot Pain: If you get shooting pains and muscle spasms in your feet on a regular basis, add wheat germ oil to your daily diet. You can use the oil as salad dressing or you can take wheat germ capsules. Start with 500 units a day and gradually work your way up. By the end of two weeks, you should have relief from the pain.

Softening Tough Feet: The soles of the feet have the body's thickest skin. To help soften and soothe this rough, tough area, get a big, juicy lemon and cut it in half the long way. Take plastic shoeboxes and divide the squeezed juice of the lemon into them. (See HEALTHFUL AND HELPFUL HINTS on how to get the most juice out of a lemon.) Cup each half of lemon on each of your heels. Put your feet into the boxes that way and add enough warm water to cover your feet. Stay like that for fifteen minutes, then rinse your feet in warm water and dry them thoroughly. You should notice a difference immediately.

Toughening Tender Feet: Each of us has out-of-town friends who are used to *driving* from place to place. When they visit New York, we shlep them around town by foot, and by the end of the day they're begging for mercy. We finally found a remedy to help toughen up their soles—

Get two plastic shoeboxes and in each put one tablespoon of alum (available at drugstores) and ½ gallon of cold water. Soak your feet in this solution for fifteen minutes after breakfast, after dinner, and right before bed.

Continue doing it for as many days as it takes to walk without pain from those tender soles.

Cracked Heels: See "urine" remedy for athlete's foot.

Weather-Related Cold Feet: To keep your feet warm in freezing weather, sprinkle a little cayenne pepper in your socks. It's an old skier's trick, but you don't have to be an old skier to use it.

Warning: The cayenne pepper will make your socks turn red. That red doesn't wash out completely. Cayenne will also make your feet red, but that should wash off completely, or watch our faces turn red.

Circulation-Related Cold Feet: For this remarkable Asian remedy you'll need ginger root, mustard powder, a grater, food processor or juicer, cheesecloth, and plastic wrap.

Make ginger juice by grating or food processing one ounce of fresh ginger root. Spoon the ground pulp into cheesecloth and squeeze out the juice into a little saucer, or put the ginger root through a juicer. Next, mix the juice with two teaspoons of mustard powder. Smear the soles of your cold feet with the mixture and then wrap the plastic wrap around each foot. Stay that way for fifteen minutes. Your feet should feel toasty warm. After you repeat the treatment for a week— seven days in a row—cold feet may no longer be a problem . . . just a memory.

Or: Take a half cup of kosher (or coarse) salt and add enough olive oil to make it into a paste consistency. For ten minutes, vigorously rub your feet with the mixture, making sure you give equal time to all the parts of your feet. In your bathtub, rinse your feet with warm water and then with cool water. Dry them with a rough towel. Your feet should feel *charged* and your circulation should be stimulated.

Toes—Tingling and Numbness: These symptoms can be indications of a vitamin B-6 deficiency. Take 50 mgs of B-6 daily and the tingling and numbness should disappear within a month.

CORN REMEDIES

Q: What's the difference between an oak tree and a tight shoe?

A: An oak tree makes acorns; a tight shoe makes corns ache.

Not funny? Neither are corns. Here are remedies—

• Before bedtime, rub the corn with either castor oil, wheat germ oil, the oil from a vitamin E capsule, or a vitamin A capsule. Do it for a few minutes, then let it sink in for the next few minutes. Finally, put a sock on that foot and go to sleep. Do this every night for a couple of weeks and you should get rid of the corn.

• Find a slim lemon and at bedtime cut out a dime-sized piece of peel from the top and insert the toe that has the corn into that opening. Put a sock on top of it and keep it on overnight. If the entire lemon on your toe is ungainly, use a wedge of lemon, or just the peel—the white side against the corn—and a Band-Aid. Do it every night until you're cornless.

•   In the morning, put a small onion in white vinegar. At bedtime, cut a piece out of the vinegar-soaked onion and put it on the corn, keeping it in place with a Band-Aid. Leave it on overnight. In the A.M., the corn may be ripe enough to remove.

Yes, this remedy has been known to work after only one application. If it doesn't, repeat the procedure the following day.

Sweaty, Smelly Feet: Drown four tea bags in a quart of just-boiled water and let them steep for fifteen minutes. Then divide the strong tea into two plastic shoeboxes and add enough cool water to make it possible to put your feet in without burning them. Soak your feet for a half hour. Do this twice a day for at least a week, and you should notice a difference, thanks to "tannin," a drying substance in tea.

Heel Spurs: Gemologist Joyce Kaessinger had a heel spur. She could hardly walk and was in constant excruciating pain.

Everything she read in medical articles or was told by a podiatrist agreed that "heel spurs are forever."

Joyce believes that whatever comes can also go and she started working with crystals.

The crystals she used were: green tourmaline, black tourmaline, smoky quartz, aventurine, and hematite. (All are inexpensive stones that are available at crystal shops.)

At night, following her intuition, she would select a few stones and tape them to the bottom of her foot and sleep that way. During the day, she would also lie on the floor and have those stones pointed at her heel while she meditated. She also said an affirmation: "I can walk comfortably for as long and as far as I desire."

In about two weeks there was a big difference. Joyce was able to walk. And not long after that, the spur completely disappeared.

Joyce feels it's important to continue using the stones and affirmation to some degree, even after you're all better.

𝒮 **Affirmation:** For all of the above foot problems, you can use Joyce Kaessinger's affirmation in the "heel spur" remedy, or you can repeat the following affirmation at least twenty times, any time you feel pain in your feet—

Walking through life with ease, I advance and grow and keep step with the world.

Fungus Among Us: Take zinc tablets, 15 mgs, three a day, to help get rid of fingernail fungus. Also, eat foods rich in zinc: raw pumpkin seeds, sunflower seeds, mushrooms, and whole grains. Zinc is also known to make white spots on fingernails disappear.

Warning: Prolonged use of zinc can cause copper deficiency. Consult with your health professional for guidance.

Vitamin E is also effective in clearing up fungus on fingernails and dry, rough, itchy skin around fingernails. Puncture a vitamin E capsule and squeeze out the oil on the problem area. Do it at least twice a day. Also, take one 400 IU capsule of vitamin E daily.

Brittle or Damaged Nails: Cut a piece of onion and rub it on your fingernails. Do it after every meal. It has nothing to do with eating—it's just that you should do this three times a day, and by assigning specific times, chances are you'll do it consistently.

Since brittle nails may be caused by iron deficiency (especially in women), add leafy green vegetables, raisins, whole grains, and fruit to your daily diet.

Taking two Evening Primrose Oil capsules (500 mgs) a day can soften your nails and do wonderful things for your skin and hair, too. Evening Primrose Oil is available at health food stores. Bring your charge card; it's quite expensive. EPO has GLA (gamma-linoleic acid), an unusual and beneficial fatty acid that most of us hardly get in our normal diet. When taking EPO, be patient. It may take up to two months to get results.

Splitting Fingernails: Eat a half-dozen raw almonds daily. It's a good source of protein, vitamins, and nutrients, plus linoleic acid that helps prevent nails from splitting. As with most of the nail remedies, it takes a while before the improvement shows.

Nail Strengthener: Steep one tablespoon of horsetail (available at health food stores) in a cup of just-boiled water. When it's cool enough to the touch, strain it and dunk your fingers in the liquid for fifteen minutes. Do this every day and give it a month or two to see an improvement.

When You Hammer the Wrong Nail: Ouch! Immediately dip your hammered fingernail in ice-cold water. It will numb the pain, keep down the swelling, and minimize the soreness. It may also prevent the nail from turning black, but we give no guarantees on this. (See BRUISES for a slammed finger or toe.)

About Nail Polish: Before polishing your fingernails, wipe the unpolished nails with white vinegar, then polish. Priming with vinegar should make your manicure last longer.

If you do your nails with nail enamel, chances are you also use acetone nail polish remover. To help prevent your nails from drying out, add about a half-dozen drops of castor oil to the bottle of nail polish remover.

The liver produces bile. The gallbladder, the liver's downstairs neighbor, stores the bile and releases it to dissolve fats. Are you wondering why I'm telling you all this?

Well, you should know that if you have sharp pains—like severe gas pains—under your right rib cage, it could mean that you have gallstones.

Have your condition medically diagnosed. While you're deciding on your plan of action, you might want to try one of these remedies—with your doctor's permission and supervision, of course.

GALLSTONE REMOVERS

• The common ingredient in almost all the gallstone remedies we've collected is olive oil. Olive oil seems to open the bile ducts, encouraging the stones to move along and out. Listen to your inner voice (and your doctor) to guide you to the method that will work best for you.

Lie down on the floor and slowly sip half a cup of warm pure virgin olive oil. If necessary, do it again in another eight hours. During this process, you might want to tape a piece of sugilite to the painful area. According to gemologist Joyce Kaessinger, sugilite is the gem that will help you let go of what's *galling* you.

• Daily, before breakfast, take two tablespoons of pure virgin olive oil, *followed* by half a cup of grapefruit juice or *in* the juice. Gradually increase the amount of oil and juice until you're up to a quarter of a cup of olive oil in a glass of grapefruit juice. You should get results within a month.

- Drink one quart of apple juice every day for five days, while eating light, sensible meals. On the sixth day, drink a quart of apple juice throughout the day, omit the evening meal, and, at six P.M., take one tablespoon of Epsom salts with half a cup of water. At eight P.M., take another tablespoon of Epsom salts with half a cup of water. Then at ten P.M. combine four ounces of pure virgin olive oil with four ounces of fresh lemon juice and drink it down. Within the next twenty-four hours, you should get rid of the gallstones. If you do all that, you *deserve* to get rid of the gallstones.

- "Take a teaspoon of fiddle rosin, put it in a tablespoon, and add jelly or syrup to fill up the tablespoon. That'll make the rosin edible. Swallow it down and, before you can say 'Geronimo,' your gallstone will high-tail it out of there."

Those are the words of a woman who called in to share this remedy with us when we were on a radio show. She told us she was brought up with Cherokee Indians and learned all this good stuff from them. Incidentally, she knows for sure that this remedy works . . . at least it worked for her.

Rosin is made of resin derived from the sap of various pine trees. You can buy it at music stores that sell string instruments.

Important: *These gallbladder remedies should be used only with your doctor's approval and under his/her close supervision.*

Sluggish Gallbladder: If your doctor's diagnosis is "sluggish gallbladder," clean out that slothful gallbladder by drinking at least seven cups of camomile tea a day for seven days. Prepare it by steeping one teaspoon of camomile in a cup of just-boiled water. After ten minutes, strain, add the juice of half a lemon, and drink.

The vitamin C from the lemon seems to add to and intensify the cleansing power of the camomile.

Be sure to get your doctor's approval before starting this cleansing treatment.

Prevention: Do not eat fatty foods—that means foods that are fried, rich desserts, fatty meats, and high-fat dairy products.

Drink lots of water and pure juices. Eat whole grains, fruits, vegetables, and if you must eat meat make sure it's lean. Boil, broil, and steam foods that you can't eat raw.

✍ **Affirmation:** While we've refrained from reporting the psychological reasons for physical manifestations, we're making an exception here, since the English language has done it for us. Take a look at your life and recognize all the things that are going on that *gall* you and acknowledge all the people you have to deal with who *gall* you. You're probably not allowing yourself to get pleasure from the everyday things in your life. Repeat the following affirmation at least fifteen times, first thing in the morning, last thing at night, and every time you walk through a doorway—

My life is a happy challenge. I find pleasure in everything I do.

HAIR

A little less than seventy percent of the American population has dark hair; only fifteen percent are blond. Is that why this country isn't having much fun?

About sixty-five percent of us have straight hair, while twenty-five percent have wavy hair, leaving only ten percent with hair that's curly.

On the average, hair grows half an inch each month—a little less in February, of course. Your hair grows fastest when you're in love, probably because your hormones are jumping for joy.

The average person loses about seventy hairs a day—more if you are sick, anemic, malnourished, or the love of your life leaves you.

Talk about losing your hair . . . One out of every five men will not lose their hair, while one out of every five men will start to lose their hair at a rapid pace in their twenties. The remaining three out of the five will get bald slowly.

It is said that the more hair a man has on his chest when he's thirty, the less hair he'll have on his head by the time he reaches forty. The hormones that are responsible for chest hair also cause male pattern baldness.

Statistics are interesting, but they aren't going to help you take care of your hair. These suggestions may—

DANDRUFF CHASERS

• Grate one ounce of fresh ginger root and take an ounce of camomile flowers (available at health food stores) and tie them into a piece of cheesecloth. Put the cheesecloth pouch in a gallon of spring water and boil it for ten minutes. When the liquid cools, pour it into bottles. Label and seal them.

To use it, after shampooing, massage one-half to one ounce into your hair. No need to rinse.

• If you have dandruff, get an aloe vera plant. The night before you're going to shampoo your hair, snip off a piece of the lowest leaf of the aloe plant. Peel off the skin of the leaf and squeeze the gel on your hair and scalp. Wrap your head in a bandanna and sleep that way. Next morning when you wash your hair, don't use shampoo. Foam up the aloe gel. It's good for your hair and can get rid of your dandruff quickly.

• Saturate your scalp and hair with warm apple cider vinegar. Cover your head with a shower cap and stay that way for an hour. Then rinse your hair with plain water. Do this twice a week until the dandruff is gone.

• Warm an ounce of peanut oil, or however much it takes for you to massage it into your scalp. Then follow that with fresh lemon juice. After keeping the oil and lemon on your head for fifteen minutes, shampoo it out. Since the strong chemicals in shampoo can cause dandruff, read labels and buy a mild, health food store shampoo.

For Healthy Hair: Include seaweed in your daily diet. It can make a major difference in your energy level, sexual desire, nervous system, digestive system, mental stress, sensory receptiveness, memory, aches and pains, oh yes, and help give you healthy hair.

Try different kinds of seaweed—dulse, kelp, hijiki, arame, wakame, nori—and discover the ones you like best. Find a macrobiotic restaurant in your area, or get a good cookbook and experiment.

If you just can't develop a taste for seaweed, you can always take it in capsule form.

For a Shinier and Fuller Head of Hair: Take a daily dose of bee pollen (available at most health food stores or check our RESOURCES). Start with a few granules daily for a few days, and if you don't have an allergic reaction, slowly increase the amount to a quarter-teaspoon a day. Slowly work your way up to a tablespoon of bee pollen daily.

For Shiny Hair and Gray Prevention: This remedy is not for everyone. It's only for those who know they can do it safely, carefully, and painlessly.

At least once a day, do a head stand. While you're in that position, gently and carefully massage your head on the floor. It is said to give you shiny hair, help prevent your hair from turning gray—and clean your floor at the same time!

When you first start this yoga exercise, do it for a very short length of time—a minute. As you feel more comfortable and confident in that position, gradually increase the number of minutes you stand on your head.

To Give Dark Hair a Shine: Prepare strong rosemary tea with a heaping tablespoon of rosemary (available at health food stores) in a pint of just-boiled water. Cover and let it steep for fifteen minutes. Strain and take the liquid with you into the shower. Shampoo your hair, rinse it with plain water and then rinse it again with the rosemary tea. (This should not be used on light or gray hair.)

To Soften Coarse Hair: Shampoo and towel-dry your hair. Then take a pint of plain yogurt and glop it on your hair, making sure it gets evenly distributed. Stay that way for fifteen minutes before rinsing out the yogurt with tepid water.

To Condition Hair: Spread mayonnaise on your hair and scalp, wrap your head in a towel, and let it stay that way for a half-hour. Then wash it out.

If you have an overripe banana hanging around and/or a squishy old avocado, mix the meats together and spread it on your hair and scalp. To avoid being attacked by fruit flies, wrap your head in a towel and stay that way for a half hour. When shampooing hair clean, take precautions not to clog up the drain in the bathtub, shower, or sink. "Hair catchers" are available at hardware stores.

For Split and Broken Ends: Gently comb a half-cup of warm castor oil or olive oil through your hair, making sure the oil reaches the ends. With the oil in place, wrap your head in a hot, wrung-out towel and stay that way for a half hour. Then add one egg yolk to your shampoo and wash your hair. Add a half-cup of apple cider vinegar to a gallon of water and make that your final rinse.

Hair-Setting Lotion: This Bud's for you—if it's gone flat and you need a setting lotion. Just comb any gone-flat beer through your hair and you're set . . . well, almost. The beer smell will disappear in less time than it takes to drink a three-pack.

Make Your Own Natural Hair Spray: Take a large lemon or two small ones, cut them into small chunks, and put the chunks in a glass or enamel sauce pan. Add two cups of water and bring it to a boil. As soon as it starts to boil, lower the flame and cook until the liquid cooks down to half the amount—it should take about fifteen to twenty minutes. Next, strain out the liquid. While you're doing that, you may want to press down on the lemon chunks to make sure all the juice is out of 'em. Put the *lemon hair spray* in a spray container and refrigerate it. If you don't use it often, put one ounce of vodka in it as a preservative.

HAIR LOSS PREVENTION

If your hair is thinning, and you are sure you are not among the ninety percent who can attribute it to hereditary factors, these suggestions may help—

• Sulfur is a mineral that nourishes scalp follicles. Eat foods rich in sulfur—cabbage, brussels sprouts, kale, watercress, turnips, cauliflower, parsnips, raspberries, and cranberries. It's best to eat the fruits and vegetables raw; second best is steamed.

Also take a B-complex vitamin. The combination of the two (sulfur-filled foods and B vitamins) should make for healthier hair and more of it.

• An Asian remedy calls for boiling one pound of snails in water. Once the water cools, wash your hair with it. It's supposed to prevent hair loss. Well, maybe you lose your hair, but at a snail's pace.

• Drink barley water on a daily basis. To prepare it, put two ounces of barley in a pot with six cups of water. Boil it down to half the amount of water. Strain and drink. (Add honey only if you need to make it more palatable.)

If the thinning of your hair has given you an ulcer, the barley water will take care of that, too!

• You might want to try washing your head with sage tea every day. Prepare the tea by using two tablespoons of sage in a pint of just-boiled water. Strain and drench your scalp with the liquid. They say it may stop your hair from falling out. (Don't ask us who "they" is.)

Grow Hair Back: There are two versions of this Chinese remedy. Each of them includes fresh ginger root, and each should be done on a daily basis.

Version #1: Finely grate a chunk of ginger and warm it just a little. Then spread it on the bald area and cover it with a shower cap for a half-hour before washing it off.

Version #2: Juice ginger (grate it or put it through a food processor and squeeze it through cheesecloth) and add alcohol—one part ginger to ten parts alcohol. Dip a cottonball in the solution and massage the bald area with it. After a half hour, rinse the head with tepid water.

❧ Hay Fever and Other Allergies ❧

What we have come to know as "hay fever" is, in most cases, an allergy to pollen and mold spores in the air. In the spring there's pollen from trees and grass; starting in mid-August, there's pollen from ragweed and other weeds, along with mold spores from barley, wheat, and corn (especially in the Midwest).

The pollen count is highest from sunrise to ten A.M., so stay indoors during those hours as much as possible.

If you have a lawn, keep your grass real short—no more than an inch high. It will limit your exposure to grass pollen.

Protection and Prevention: Wear a mask over your mouth and nose when you do gardening and avoid tons of pollen. Masks are available at hardware stores. Indoors, wear the mask whenever you vacuum, to avoid inhaling the dust that gets churned up.

Here are some more suggestions for pre-season immunization that we hope will prevent problems. (If it's too late for this year, check out the remedies that can help quell an attack.)

• Four months before the hay fever season starts, build an immunity to airborne pollen by taking bee pollen. If you don't have a local beekeeper, you can get bee pollen at health food stores or check the RESOURCES section for our recommendations.

You must start real slow to make sure you're not allergic to bee pollen. Take three little granules of bee pollen the first day. If you have no reaction, good. Continue to take three granules for a few days. Then take ten granules for a few days. Slowly, *slowly,* work your way up to a quarter-teaspoon, then a half-teaspoon, three-quarters of a teaspoon, and—the big time—a teaspoon a day.

You can put it in anything—juice, cereal—or dissolve it in your mouth and/or just swallow it.

It's an amazingly effective remedy. Then again, bee pollen is one of nature's perfect foods, containing all the necessary nutrients to sustain life. It's also one of the few things that cannot be duplicated in a laboratory.

• A daily cup of fenugreek seed tea (available at health food stores), starting three months *before* the hay fever season, can desensitize you. The name "fenugreek" means "Greek hay."

• Two months before hay fever month rolls around, take brewer's yeast tablets. Read the label for the recommended dosage.

Immunity Boosters: Red clover blossoms (available at health food stores) were a favorite of medieval herbalists and are now gaining popularity again. It's no wonder. Three or four cups of red clover tea a day can help build an immunity to allergies.

Daily doses of garlic and horseradish can help build your resistance to allergies. Finely mince a clove of garlic and put it in orange juice or some water and drink it down. Add a quarter-teaspoon of horseradish to vegetable juice or mix it in a salad. Both are strong and may take getting used to. If they help you breathe easier, minimize your allergy symptoms, and maybe even immunize yourself against allergies, start getting used to 'em!

Relief Is on the Way: I've gotten instant relief from a hay fever attack by chewing a one-inch square of honeycomb (available at health food stores). It's delicious. You swallow the honey and continue chewing the waxy gum for about ten minutes. Be sure that the honeycomb is from your area of the country—the closer the better.

Nettle, a common plant, also known as stinging nettle, seems to act as a natural antihistamine and offers quick relief from a hay fever attack. According to Dr. Andrew Weil, a freeze-dried extract of the leaves taken in capsules is best. To control symptoms, take one or two capsules every two to four hours.

Breathe Easier: Slice an onion right before you eat dinner and let it sit in a glass of water. When you're ready for bed, drink the onion water. It should help you fall asleep and breathe easier while you sleep.

Stuffed Nose: When your nose is stuffed, rub your ears vigorously until they feel as though they're burning. For some odd reason, it should clear up the stuffiness.

Aromatherapy: Hyssop, lavender, or camomile oils are said to relieve hay fever symptoms. When you have a runny nose, teary eyes, and that stuffed-up feeling, put a drop or two of any of the above oils on the inside of your wrist or on a handkerchief, and take a whiff every few minutes.

Chihuahua Cure: We received a letter from a woman who told us about three different cases that she knew of where Chihuahuas somehow rid their owners of severe allergies. The most dramatic of the three stories was about a young girl who had been suffering with hay fever for several years and had tried everything. As a last resort, her uncle bought her a Chihuahua. The family thought he was crazy, but it was an adorable little pet and his niece was happy to have this new friend. The bottom line is, the last hay fever attack the young girl ever had was the day *before* she got the dog.

Food Allergies: The foods that most often cause allergic reactions are: eggs, corn, cow's milk, wheat, citrus fruit, tomatoes, cane sugar, seafood, nuts, and chocolate. Talk about chocolate . . . If you're allergic to it and really want to continue eating it, try *white* chocolate. It doesn't have theobromine, which may be the substance in *dark* chocolate that causes your allergic reaction.

Ragweed Allergy Symptoms: If your hay fever is due to ragweed, you may experience the identical misery-making symptoms after eating cantaloupe, watermelon, honeydew, zucchini, or cucumber. These fruits and vegetables have extraordinarily similar allergy-producing proteins to ragweed, so avoid them.

Shrimp Alert: If you're allergic to shrimp, don't eat them. You didn't need us to tell you that. What you may not know is that you shouldn't even go into the kitchen when they're being prepared. Breathing in the steam that filters out into the air while shrimp are boiling can be enough to trigger an allergic reaction.

Pesticides and Preservatives: If your allergies are caused by pesticides or preservatives on fruits and vegetables, eat foods rich in selenium: bran, broccoli, onions, tuna in water, tomatoes, and Brazil nuts. (See HEALTHFUL AND HELPFUL HINTS for ways to clean produce.) Supplement your diet with selenium tablets (available at health food stores) and follow the recommended dosage on the bottle. Selenium may also help protect you from pollution in the air.

Nickel Allergy: An allergy to nickel is the most common contact allergy among women. The metal pins worn for the first three to six weeks after ears are pierced contain minute quantities of nickel.

People who have their ears pierced with more than one hole in each ear have twice as many allergies. See EARS/Referral for a contact for hypoallergenic earrings.

Incidentally, nickel is found in high quality gold, silver, and platinum as well as cheaper costume varieties. That nickel can trigger an allergy to metal that makes you vulnerable when you wear any kind of jewelry or even metal buttons, snaps, eyeglass frames, wrist watches, and zippers.

Fabric Allergies: If you have a sneaking suspicion that you're allergic to a specific fabric, take a piece of that fabric—a swatch will do—put it in a jar with the lid on, and leave it in the sun for five hours. Then open the jar and inhale the air in the jar. If you sneeze, wheeze, turn red, perspire, or manifest any allergic reaction, guess what . . . you're allergic to that fabric.

𝒮 **Affirmation:** Repeat this affirmation at least ten times, starting first thing in the morning, every time you leave a place, including your home, and every time you enter a new place, including your car or public transportation, your office, a supermarket—wherever. Then, repeat it another ten times last thing at night.

Everything is happening for my good. I am safe and I am free to enjoy life.

REFERRAL

For a free packet of information, call Asthma and Allergy Foundation of America at 202/466-7643.

HEADACHES

A headache happens when small blood vessels within the skull open up and cause increased pressure. That pressure is responsible for the pain we know as a headache.

There are tension headaches, sinus headaches, hangover headaches, headaches caused by overeating, constipation, cold/flu, eyestrain, allergies, and everything else you can think of. Ice cream!—some people even get headaches when they eat very cold ice cream. That's an easy headache to prevent. Don't eat very cold ice cream. Another no-no: Refrain from chewing chewing gum. The constant sameness of movement can stress muscles, which in turn can cause a tension headache.

HEADACHE REMEDIES

Thanks to television commercials, we now know what a headache looks like. Thanks to the following remedies, you may be able to get rid of a headache by the time you can say, "acetylsalicylic acid."

• Make a poultice of fresh grated horseradish in cheesecloth and put the poultice on the back of your neck. While you're at it, put two smaller horseradish poultices in each bend of your elbows. Keep poultices on for at least thirty minutes or until the headache disappears.

• Get in the swing of things with Li Shou, which is Chinese for "hand swinging." By flailing your arms vigorously, you make more blood flow to your arms and less blood flow to your head. That should help reduce the swelling of the vessels in the skull that caused your headache in the first place.

- Massage two drops of peppermint oil (available in health food stores) on your temples. If you have particularly sensitive skin, do not use peppermint oil directly on your skin. Also, if possible, relax in a hot bath while drinking a cup of peppermint tea.

- If you have a headache over one eye, take a clothespin and put it on the lobe of the ear that's on the same side as the headache. We've gotten reports that this clothespin remedy works fast—and that isn't just a line!

- The University of California's headache specialists feel that tension headaches are caused by improper blood supply to the brain, starting from tension at the base of the neck and in the shoulders. Their treatment of choice is massage to relax the tense muscles. That's what friends are for.

- Every time we visited our grandmother, she was wearing a head band. It was my grandfather's white handkerchief, dipped in vinegar, wrung out, rolled up, and tied around her forehead. Lydia was ten years old before she realized that *Bubby* wasn't a Native American . . . or Willie Nelson in drag: Our grandmother used to get headaches and the vinegar head band worked for her.

Koreans use a similar remedy. They tie a bandanna (without the vinegar) tightly around their heads, right over the eyebrows.

Or, forget the bandanna and stick with the vinegar. Mix two tablespoons of apple cider vinegar with two teaspoons of honey in a glass of water, drink it slowly, and get results within a half-hour.

Acupressure: Place your third finger an inch above the bridge of your nose in the center of your forehead. Without lifting your finger, massage the area in a circular motion. Do it for seven to ten minutes. If it doesn't drive the headache out by the end of ten minutes, try something else.

Gem Therapy: Amethysts are the tranquilizer of the mineral world.

When you have a tension headache, lie down and gently rub the smooth side of an amethyst on your forehead. Rubbing a stone activates its healing vibration. Once it's activated, let it rest on your forehead while you relax. You may also want to repeat the affirmation at the end of this chapter.

Visualization: According to Dr. Gerald Epstein, psychiatrist, imagery expert, and author of *Healing Visualizations* (Bantam Books, 1989), headaches are characteristically related to one's emotional state. Tension headaches involve worry, and mirror the tension you feel in your life.

The remedy? Have your secretary hold all calls, put a DO NOT DISTURB sign on your door, sit in a comfortable chair, and follow these instructions in what Dr. Epstein calls the "Lake of the Brain" exercise to visualize away your tension headache. Do the exercise as needed, every five to ten minutes, for up to three minutes each time.

> Close your eyes and breathe out three times. Look down at the top of your head. Lift off the top of your skull as if you were removing the top of the shell of a soft-boiled egg. Look inside. See the fluid of your brain and the moving nerve fibers that look like water plants underneath. See the fluid draining out of your head completely and sense and feel the tension relieved at the base of your skull and the back of your neck, sensing the fluid moving down the spinal column to the base. See fresh fluid moving up the spinal column, through the neck, and filling your skull, seeing through the clean, clear liquid to the nerve fibers below. Feel and sense the flow of fresh blood through your neck and down into the rest of your body. Put on the top of your skull, breathe out once, and open your eyes.

Morning Headaches: If you wake up with a headache, it may be that your bedroom has stale air. The room should always have circulating air at night.

Weekend Headaches: If you're a coffee drinker who goes to work during the week and gets headaches at home on the weekend, listen up.

Chances are, you have your first cup of coffee before you leave for work in the morning. Then you probably have your second cup an hour or so after arriving at work. When you're at home over the weekend and don't have to get up as early as you do for work, you may have your first cup of coffee later than usual. The difference of those few hours can cause caffeine withdrawal and the dilation of the blood vessels that increase pressure in the skull—and poof!—a headache.

Either cut out coffee completely, or, on the weekend, have your first cup at the same time as when you go to work.

TEMPORAL HEADACHES

A temporal headache is experienced as that "pounding in my head" where there is great pressure felt at both sides of the head in the region of the temporal bones (your temples). It can arise when you do not allow yourself to say what you feel.

Visualization: According to Dr. Gerald Epstein, the emotional state that's characteristically related to temporal headaches involves rage.

Dr. Epstein's visualization for temporal headaches is called "The Silver Band." Find a comfortable chair where you will not be disturbed and do this exercise every five to ten minutes, for one to two minutes, until the headache disappears.

Close your eyes. Breathe out three times and imagine a silver band stretched tightly across your skull from temporal bone to temporal bone and flaring out slightly at the ends as it lies on the bones.

See and sense the band tightening around your skull, with the ends pressing against the temporal bones and then quickly releasing; the band and ends squeeze once again and then release quickly; and again a third time. Then open your eyes, knowing that the pain has gone.

MIGRAINE HEADACHES

According to neurologist Dr. Lawrence Newman, who is in charge of the Headache Unit at New York's Montefiore Medical Center, half of all migraines are caused by food allergies. Any food can be the culprit, but most common are aged cheeses, chocolate, citrus fruit, and red wine. Sodium nitrates (found in frankfurters, ham, bacon, lunch meats) and other food additives such as MSG are also responsible for many migraines. Consult with a health professional to determine whether or not you have a food allergy that's causing your migraines.

A few interesting-but-useless facts:

• Allergies and migraines are more prevalent among left-handed people.

• "Migraine" comes from a Latin word that means "pain in half the head," although a migraine can occur in more or less than half the head.

• Seventy-five percent of migraine sufferers are women, not that you'd know it from this list of male victims: Edgar Allan Poe, Rudyard Kipling, Leo Tolstoy, Lewis Carroll, Frederic Chopin, Peter Ilyich Tchaikovsky, Sigmund Freud, Charles Darwin, Julius Caesar, Peter the Great, Thomas Jefferson, Ulysses S. Grant, Karl Marx, Woody Allen, and Kareem Abdul-Jabbar.

Since misery likes company, we thought that prestigious list would make you feel better. To make you feel a whole lot better, you might want to try the following remedies:

MIGRAINE REMEDIES

• Put your feet in a basin of hot water and an ice pack on the back of your neck. This remedy came to us from a California screenwriter, and screenwriters know from headaches.

• Ice packs on the head and neck *without* the feet in hot water (see above) seem to help some migraine sufferers.

• We realize that this book is not a products catalog, but when it comes to pain as nasty as migraine or tension headaches, we feel compelled to share something that's safe, easy to use, proven successful in eighty percent of the cases, and reasonably priced at under fifty dollars. It's called the Headache ICE-PILLO, a horseshoe-shaped cushion with a frozen soft gel pack insert that wraps around the back of the neck and supports the head. The cold gel conforms to the muscles and blood vessels in the area of the neck that contributes to headaches. Using the pillow at the first dull pain of a migraine can prevent it from happening, or can make the pain fade a lot faster than usual.

Invented by Dr. Lee Kudrow of the California Medical Clinic for Headache in Encino, California, this pillow has undergone extensive testing with impressive results. Four out of five people tested got rid of the migraines.

For details about the Headache ICE-PILLO, see Referral. Incidentally, you do not have to mention our names or this book. We have absolutely nothing to do with the sale of this product.

• Take a slice of watermelon, eat the meat, and bind the rind! Make sure the rind stretches across your forehead to your temples and hold it in place with a handkerchief or Ace bandage. While waiting for the watermelon rind to draw out the pain, you might want to repeat the "Tension Headache" affirmation given at the end of this chapter.

• Eat a dozen raw almonds or smear an eighth-teaspoon of almond oil on a slice of bread and eat it slowly.

• Caffeine seems to constrict the blood vessels in the skull. That generally reduces the pain of a migraine. Prepare a very strong cup of Chinese black tea and sip it slowly for fast relief.

Visualization: Dr. Gerald Epstein says that migraine headaches most often involve anger. His visualization exercise for migraines is called "Open Eyes." Relax in a comfortable chair in a quiet place, and do the exercise as needed when headache occurs, for two to three minutes at a time.

> With your eyes open, look up and out to the side
> of the headache for two to three minutes steadily.
> Then return to your normal gaze.

Migraine Prevention: The herb feverfew has a centuries-old reputation as a remarkable migraine headache remedy. It's available in capsule form at health food stores. Follow the dosage on the label.

Or drink a cup of yarrow tea daily. If you buy the loose herb (available at health food stores), rather than teabags, use a heaping teaspoon in a cup of just-boiled water. Strain and drink slowly. Yarrow is an odd-tasting herb. Give it time—it'll grow on you.

For women only: Get pregnant. For some unknown reason, women don't have migraines while they're pregnant.

✌ **Affirmation:** Repeat this affirmation at least fifteen times, first thing in the morning, last thing at night, and at the first sign of tension.

I am wonderful! I love and appreciate myself.

REFERRAL

For information about The Headache ICE-PILLO, and ICE-BAND, which are FDA-listed, call 800/992-PAIN.

Antibiotics: If you are put on antibiotics, be sure to take acidophilus (available at health food stores). The antibiotics have no discretion; they destroy the good as well as the bad bacteria. Acidophilus replaces the beneficial bacteria. Capsules should have one to two billion viable acidophilus cells. No, you don't have to count them. Read the label carefully.

Important: Take acidophilus right after you've eaten and at least two hours before or two hours after you take an antibiotic. That way you won't make the antibiotic crazy going after the acidophilus' beneficial bacteria.

An Apple (or Two) a Day: Researchers studied students who ate two apples a day and compared them to students who didn't eat any apples. The apple eaters were less stressed, had fewer headaches, and were more emotionally stable. Apple eaters also seem to have clearer skin, fewer colds, and are not as troubled by arthritis.

Avocados—When Are They Ripe?: Give it the five-finger test. Let an avocado rest in the palm of one hand and put the fingers of your other hand on the side of an avocado. Gently press in. If it feels as though the pit inside is detaching itself from the meat of the fruit, then the avocado is ripe.

Band-Aid Removal: Soak a cotton ball with vegetable oil or baby oil and dab it all over the Band-Aid. The Band-Aid will peel off painlessly.

Or, let a hair dryer blow warm air on the Band-Aid for a minute or two. The heat will melt the sticky stuff, making it possible to peel without pain.

Bioflavonoids: You've probably heard the word "bioflavonoids" in television commercials, but do you know what they do and how to get them?

What they do is promote the absorption of vitamin C and they reinforce the walls of small blood vessels that deliver nutrients to individual cells.

You get bioflavonoids from the white layer of skin that you usually peel off citrus fruits and throw away. Do not be so quick to throw it away. Instead, eat some of that bioflavonoid white skin.

Bleeding: While waiting for professional medical attention, there is a simple way to help stop bleeding most places on the body. Measure five inches down from the knees, on the inside of both legs, and press in for a few minutes—until the bleeding stops.

Cold Weather Dressing: Opt for mittens rather than gloves. They'll keep your hands warmer.

Another way to keep your hands warm, and feet too, is by wearing a hat.

Thin layers of clothing will keep you warmer than one heavy layer. Your body heats the air that's between the layers and insulates you from the cold.

People think a good stiff drink will warm them. *Wrong!* Alcohol dilates blood vessels and that results in a *loss* of heat.

Using Computers: The National Institute of Occupational Safety and Health recommends that you—

• Position the screen at eye level, about twenty-two to twenty-six inches away.

• Sit about arm's length from the terminal. At that distance, the electrical field is almost zero.

• Face forward and keep your neck relaxed.

• Position the keyboard so that elbows are bent at least ninety degrees and you can work without bending your wrists.

- Use a chair that supports your back, lets your feet rest on the floor or footrest, and keeps thighs parallel to the floor.

- If you can step away from the computer for fifteen minutes every hour, it can help prevent eyestrain.

Cookware Care: Recent research suggests that we need to be as concerned about using copper or ceramic cookware as the much-maligned aluminum cookware. We suggest that you avoid using aluminum or copper cookware, but if you do use them, here are ways to help minimize their harmful effects:

To prevent the leaching of aluminum from a new pot or pan, wash it with hot sudsy water and rinse. Next, fill it with water, boil for two to three minutes, then throw out that water. From then on, the aluminum should not leach into food.

As for copper cookware, some inexpensive brands have copper as the cooking surface, and that can leach out in unhealthy amounts. Copper cookware is okay, only if it has a stainless-steel cooking surface.

Worst of all is ceramic, from which lead can leach into the food it holds. Lead—even low levels of it—can be seriously toxic, especially to children. To prevent possible lead poisoning, the FDA advises against the use of ceramic cookware from China, Mexico, India, or Hong Kong. If you are using ceramic cookware, do not cook or store acidic foods like tomatoes, orange juice, or vinegar in it. And don't put ceramic in the dishwasher.

There are lead-testing kits on the market. If you have doubts about the safety of your dishes and other items in the home, especially if they're used by children, you may want to get one of the lead-testing kits on the market.

If you use castiron pots and pans for cooking, the food will absorb some of the iron and, in turn, you will, too. This is particularly beneficial for women who are menstruating and lose iron. It can, however, be harmful to people who do not need the additional iron. Know your needs and cook with caution.

"Eggs-cellent" Advice: When you buy eggs, keep them in your refrigerator in the carton they came in. If any salmonella exists, the egg section in the refrigerator door will not keep them cold enough to discourage the salmonella from multiplying, especially if the door is opened often.

• Throw out eggs that are cracked. They may be contaminated. Better safe than salmonella.

• Do not eat foods that have raw eggs in them, like hollandaise sauce and caesar salad.

• To avoid salmonella, it's eggs-tremely important to prepare them properly. The standard safe cooking times are:
Scrambled—two eggs, three minutes over low-medium fire.
Scrambled in microwave—per egg, twenty seconds on high, take out, stir, rotate cooking dish, put egg(s) back for another twenty seconds on high.
Poached—boil for five minutes.
Sunny-side-up—four minutes over low-medium fire in a covered pan (yolk should begin to thicken).
Over easy—fry three minutes on one side, two minutes on the other over low-medium fire in a covered pan.
Soft-boiled—seven minutes in boiling water.

Feet-Soaking Made Easy: We find that the best way to soak each foot comfortably is in a plastic shoebox. It's neater and more comfortable than a basin.

Garlic Smell Remover: Take the smell of garlic off your hands by rubbing celery, or tomato, or lemon on your hands.
Our favorite garlic smell remover: Pretend a piece of silverware is a bar of soap and wash your hands with it under cold water. It works like magic.

Get Well Faster: Try to imagine the smell of homemade bread just taken out of the oven. The thought alone can make you feel warm inside. The real thing, that is, the smell of freshly baked bread, is said to actually have the power to make you feel better and get better faster.
The scent of fresh eucalyptus leaves is also very healing. If you can't get the fresh leaves, use the essential oil.

Hot Weather Endurance: To stay cooler in the warmer months, take an additional 250 mgs of vitamin C every day.

Ice Pack Substitute: If you need an ice pack but don't have one, you can use a package of frozen vegetables. Rap it with a hammer to break up the clumps of veggies, making it flexible and easy to work with.

Immune System Strengtheners: The main active ingredient in aloe vera is acemannan and it's thought to bolster the immune system's effectiveness. Take an ounce of aloe vera juice before each meal daily.

• For many years, the scientific community has recognized the importance of echinacea as an herb that helps the immune system do its job. Echinacea comes in different forms—tablets, capsules, tincture. Talk to your health professional for the dosage that's appropriate for you, or follow the suggested dose on the label.

• Stepping into a cold bath or under a cold shower for a few minutes every day can improve circulation as well as the immune system.

• Eat a portion of salt-free sauerkraut every day. The raw, fermented cabbage is rich in selenium, which is known to help strengthen the immune system.

• Bee pollen, one of nature's perfect foods, can enhance immune system function. Start by taking a few granules of bee pollen a day to make sure you have no allergic reaction to it. If all is well after three days, increase the amount to a quarter-teaspoon. Gradually, over the next month or two, work your way up to three teaspoons of bee pollen throughout each day.

Leg Shaving: To prevent ingrown hairs, go with the grain and shave *down,* from your knee to your ankle. Going against the grain can cause ingrown hairs. Well, you've been lucky so far.

To prevent dry legs, throw 'way the shaving cream; lose the soap. Shave with oil instead—sesame, peanut, or sunflower oil—and have a leg up when it comes to smooth and silky skin.

Lemons—The Big Squeeze: You will get almost twice as much juice from a lemon if you squeeze it after it sits in hot water for a few minutes. Also, roll the lemon around on your counter several times before squeezing.

To get the juice without the pits, wrap a wet piece of cheesecloth around the cut side of the lemon and strain the juice as you squeeze it out.

Liquid Foods as Cleansers: Cold tea is supposed to shine your mirror. I just tried it with a cold, wet peppermint tea bag. I wet the mirror with it, then wiped it with a paper towel, and it's as clean as can be.

• Potato water is a popular old folk remedy for many ailments. If you have any doubt about its power, soak tarnished silver in potato water for a couple of hours and see how it cleans the tarnish away.

• Worcestershire sauce shines brass. I just tried it. Don't throw away your brass polish. Or, use the Worcestershire sauce *until* you get a good brass polish.

Married Men and Housework: According to a four-year study of married couples, men who did housework were healthier than those who didn't. It seems that willingness to use a little elbow grease is representative of one's ability to deal with marital strife and life's pressures. Okay, fellas, get out the vacuum!

Medicine Made Easy: If you have to take something unpleasant, whether it's an herb or a pill, numb your taste buds first by sucking on an ice cube for a couple of minutes.

If you're going to have herb tea, the heat of the tea will counteract the numbness of your tongue. In that case, just make up your mind to acquire a taste for the herb.

You know that awful feeling when a pill or capsule doesn't go down smoothly? Dr. Hans H. Neumann, Connecticut public health physician, suggests that after taking pills or capsules you follow with a bite of banana, chew it well, and swallow. He says, "The banana helps to coat the esophagus and push the pill into the stomach for quick absorption."

Dr. Ray Wunderlich, Jr. suggests liquids with texture such as tomato juice or other vegetable juices make pill-swallowing much easier. (Apple juice is problematic.)

Metal Removers: Part of the pollution we breathe every day, especially those of us who live in smoggy big and/or industrial cities, are heavy metals—cadmium, mercury, lead, copper, and more.

Vegetables that are rich in sulfur—sweet potatoes and cabbage—can help detoxify our systems of these metals. Eat them often, at least several times a week.

Microwave Warming Warning: Food should be heated to at least 165° Fahrenheit to destroy harmful bacteria.

For reheating single portions more effectively, use half the power for a longer time. While reheating large portions, stir the food a couple of times to keep uniform temperature throughout.

Moonstruck: Those stories about a full moon and how it affects us?—all true . . . so it seems.

With relation to health, if you have any existing condition, take extra good care of yourself just before and during a full moon phase. Come to think of it, you should *always* take extra good care of yourself, no matter what phase you're going through!

No Sweat: During those dog days of summer, when you have to do something physically taxing in a non-air-conditioned location, chew a chunk of honeycomb (available at health food stores). The honeycomb can actually cause a drop in body temperature, keeping you from feeling the heat.

Onion Smell Remover: See Garlic Smell Remover.

Onions Without Tears: Put onions in the freezer for twenty minutes and then you can tearlessly chop 'em, dice 'em, mince 'em, slice 'em.

Or, keep a kitchen match in your mouth—sulfur side out—while you work with onions.

Pesticide Removal for Fruits and Vegetables: Jay Kordich, known as "The Juiceman," shared with us his method of removing poisonous sprays and pesticides from produce. Fill the sink with cold water and add four tablespoons of salt and the fresh juice of half a lemon. This makes a diluted form of hydrochloric acid. Soak most fruits and vegetables five to ten minutes; soak leafy greens two to three minutes; soak strawberries, blueberries, and all other berries one to two minutes. After soaking, rinse thoroughly in plain cold water and enjoy.

An alternative to the Juiceman's method is to soak produce in a sink or basin with a quarter of a cup of white vinegar. Then, with a vegetable brush, scrub the produce under cold water. Give them a final rinse and they're ready to be eaten.

Pineapple Ripener: Usually, the bottom of the pineapple gets ripe and even overripe while the crown with its spikey leaves stays green. To remedy this, turn a pineapple upside down and keep it that way. To test for ripeness, pluck a little leaf. If it comes out easily, the pineapple is ready for eating.

Problem Solving: Laura Silva, healer, international lecturer, and seminar leader for Silva Mind Method, says you can create an ultra state of awareness by questioning yourself. As you're going to sleep and are in a completely relaxed state, ask yourself whatever it is you want answered. Laura tells you to phrase it this way, "If I knew that answer, what would it be?" Or, "If I had the solution, what would it be?" Or, "If I knew which path to take, which path would I take?"

According to Laura, when you're in a relaxed state, these questions open up your mind to creative problem solving.

Radioactivity Remover: Japanese research suggests that miso, a food condiment made from fermented soybean paste, can remove radioactive elements from the body and reduce injury caused by radiation exposure.

Miso is available at most health food stores and at Japanese groceries. If you want to know more about the benefits of miso, the different kinds of miso, and how to prepare them, you might want to read *The Book of Miso* by Shurtleff and Aoyagi (Ballantine Books, 1981).

Recycling Plastic Bags: The printing on plastic bags—like the kind with fruit printed on it that you get at the greengrocer—can contain lead. The same holds true for the printing on most plastic bags that loaves of bread are packaged in. If you use a plastic bag with printing on it, be sure the printed surface does not touch food. When you recycle the bags, don't turn them inside out. The food can absorb the lead; then the lead would be absorbed by whomever eats the food.

Ring Removal: When your finger is a little swollen and you can't take off a ring, put your hand in ice-cold water. The cold water will cause your finger to contract and the ring will come off easily.

Salad Savvy: Prepare a salad as close to mealtime as possible. The longer a salad stands, the more vitamins are lost and the less value the food has.

Salt Reducers: The National Academy of Sciences recommends staying under 1,800 mgs of sodium a day; definitely not more than 2,400 mgs.

To help you keep your sodium count down if you use canned foods—and vegetables in particular—put the contents of the can in a strainer and rinse under your cold water faucet for at least a minute. It can reduce the salt content by more than fifty percent.

At mealtimes, add salt *after* you prepare your food. That way, you'll use half as much salt without compromising taste.

Salt Substitutes: When appropriate—according to the foods or drinks being prepared—lemon juice can be used as a substitute for salt.

You can also add spice to your life with McCormick & Company's three salt-substitute recipes:

- For salads or salt shakers—
  two teaspoons thyme
  two teaspoons ground savory
  one teaspoon sage
  two teaspoons basil
  one tablespoon marjoram

- For soups, stews, poultry, or pot roast—
  one tablespoon thyme
  one teaspoon sage
  two teaspoons rosemary
  one tablespoon marjoram
- For cooked vegetables, beef, or added table seasoning—
  one teaspoon celery seeds
  one tablespoon marjoram
  one tablespoon thyme
  one tablespoon basil

Mix ingredients for the blend you choose and grind together in a blender or using a mortar and pestle. Store in a tightly covered dark glass jar, and be sure to label for which use it's intended.

Soda Pop?—Stop!: Next time you reach for a soft drink, think twice. A recent study shows that excessive consumption of soda pop can weaken bones.

REFERRAL

If you would like to know more about Silva Mind Method, there's a free Lectures Directory, telling you when and where you can attend a free lecture. For the Directory, call or write to:

Silva Mind Method
P.O. Box 2249
Laredo, Texas 78044
800/545-6463

Dr. Willis Potts, noted heart surgeon, said, "The heart is a tough organ: a marvelous mechanism that, mostly without repairs, will give valiant service up to a hundred years."

These suggestions may help rack up the hundred years:

Please check with your health professional before trying any of these self-help remedies, whether or not you have a history of heart problems.

Arteriosclerosis Prevention: Avoid animal fats. If you do eat greasy food—especially fatty meat—have raw garlic and onion, too. Or take a couple of garlic/onion pills daily. No matter how much garlic and onion you have, you still have to cut down your animal fat intake significantly to help prevent arteriosclerosis, which is specifically related to fatty deposits in the arteries.

A lot of research is now being done on walnuts and walnut oil. In the Orient, walnuts have been used for medicinal purposes for a long time. A Chinese herbalist told us that eating three walnuts a day can help prevent arteriosclerosis. Eat the walnuts along with a sensible, heart-safe diet and get regular exercise.

Heart Disease Prevention: If you like hot and spicy, this is for you. Eat two teaspoons of jalapeño pepper every day. Pepper can stimulate the body function that dissolves blood clots, thus helping to prevent heart disease.

Palpitations: Prepare a cup of rosemary tea and/or wild cherry bark tea (available at health food stores) with one teaspoon of the herb in one cup of just-boiled water. Let it steep for seven minutes. Strain and drink three cups a day for prevention; and a cup whenever the palpitations act up.

The wild cherry bark tea has the power to calm you down quickly. The rosemary tea helps strengthen the heart.

Aromatherapy for Palpitations: Relax in a warm bath to which you've added six drops of orange blossom oil, also called neroli, and available at most health food stores.

Heart Strengthening Exercise: So you want to lead a band? Good!—it's great exercise for the heart. A study concluded that orchestra conductors live seven-and-a-half years longer than the average person. It's no wonder. Conducting is a real workout that helps strengthen the heart muscle and tone the circulatory system.

Get a baton at a music shop, or use a pencil or chopstick. Select music that lights your fire. Tap the music stand—you're ready to begin.

You may need to start slowly and work your way up to ten minutes a day, or twenty minutes three times a week. Check with your doctor before you make your debut.

After a Heart Attack: Get a pet! Studies show that the majority of people who have had heart attacks and who have pets have a speedier recuperation period and a longer survival rate than people without pets.

Angina—Night Attack Prevention: Raise the head of your bed a few inches. Put wooden blocks under the legs at the head end of your bed. According to a noted cardiologist, sleeping propped up like that can help stop the nighttime angina attacks.

For Preventing an Angina Attack: If you don't have a sensitivity to iodine, and you're not on a low-salt diet, kelp capsules (available at health food stores) can be extremely beneficial. Take up to six capsules daily. Ask your health professional to help determine your dosage.

Herb for a Healthier Heart: Hawthorn berries won our heart. According to John B. Lust, naturopath, herbalist, and author, hawthorn can help regulate heart action, normalize blood pressure, is good for heart muscle weakened by age, beneficial for inflammation of the heart muscle, for arteriosclerosis, and for nervous heart problems.

You can drink hawthorn berry tea, take hawthorn (freeze-dried extract) capsules, or hawthorn tincture. Dosage depends on your condition and the medication you may or may not be taking. Talk it over with your health professional and take it with his or her supervision. You should be monitored, especially if you're on medication, because as the hawthorn improves your condition, you might be able to cut down on your medication.

Vitamin for a Healthier Heart: According to recent research, vitamin C can profoundly help prevent arterial damage which, in turn, leads to heart attacks and strokes.

Eat foods rich in vitamin C—citrus fruit and leafy green vegetables—and supplement your diet daily with at least 250 mgs of vitamin C.

Prayer for a Healthier Heart: There was a study conducted of two groups of people born into the same religion. One group of people had a firm belief in God, and practiced the traditions of their religion on a daily basis; the other was a non-practicing group. The observant group had fewer heart attacks than the non-observant group.

In analyzing these results, the researchers said, "The strong belief in a Supreme Being and the role of prayer may in themselves be protective."

♪ **Affirmation:** Repeat this affirmation twelve times, starting first thing in the morning, every time you sigh, every time you shake your head "no," and last thing at night.

I choose to love myself and my life. I find goodness and beauty all around me.

Hemorrhoids are varicose veins in or around the rectum. As you might imagine, sitting on a horse is a real pain in the anus.

Napoleon had hemorrhoids and was unable to sit on his horse to survey the battlefield and plan his next move. So he let his next-in-command do the planning from atop his steed. *Generally* speaking, the next-in-command was not as clever a military strategist as Napoleon and it didn't take long before Napoleon was defeated at Waterloo . . . and all because of his hemorrhoids.

The whole course of history could be different if Bonaparte had known about the following remedies—

HEMORRHOID REMEDIES

With a cotton swab, apply any one of the following several times throughout the day and right before bed—dampen a cotton ball with one from the list below and place it against your rectum.

- The oil from a vitamin E capsule or wheat germ oil.

- Mix a half-teaspoon of mustard powder (be sure it's *not* "hot" mustard powder) with a tablespoon of honey (raw honey is best).

- Lemon juice (yes, it might sting).

- Witch hazel, especially if there's bleeding (and yes, it might sting).

- Papaya juice (pure and additive-free). Papaya pills also have papain, papaya's healing enzyme. They're inexpensive and taste like candy. Take four *orally* after every meal.

- Aloe vera gel or juice (available at health food stores). Also take one teaspoon of the aloe *orally* after every meal.

- Make a poultice of white bread that's been dipped in egg white and place it against the rectum.

- Peel a clove of garlic and insert it in the rectum. Put in a fresh clove at bedtime, pushing it up high. To make sure it stays in overnight, you may need to cover the spot with a bandage. We've gotten a lot of positive feedback on this remedy. It's amazing what people will talk to us about these days.

Reflexology for Hemorrhoids: The back of the leg, an inch or two up from the ankle bone, is the reflex area that relates to the rectum. Gently massage that sensitive area and you may get hemorrhoidal relief.

♪ **Affirmation:** Repeat this affirmation at least twelve times, first thing in the morning, last thing at night, and throughout the day every time you sit down—

I set myself free of anger and resentment, leaving room for all the good things coming to me now.

REFERRAL

ClenZone is an appliance that attaches to the toilet seat. It has a squirter that gets you *very* clean and gives you a brief-but-soothing bath at the same time. For more details, write or call Harry Epstein at:

ClenZone
Hepp Industries, Inc.
687 Kildare Crescent
Seaford, NY 11783
516/735-0032

❧ HERPES GENITALIS ❧

Over twenty million Americans have herpes genitalis, a sexually transmitted viral infection that's painful and unpredictably recurrent. Conservatively speaking, one out of every five sexually active adults has it. So, you are not alone. Then again, if you were *alone,* maybe you wouldn't have it.

Here are not remedies, but *treatments* to make you more comfortable, to do away with the symptoms and to prevent them from returning.

Relieve the Itching: Goldenseal, a gift from the Cherokee Indians, can help relieve the itching and dry up the lesions. Buy goldenseal in powder form, add enough water to make a paste, and gently smear it on the sores.

Hasten the Healing: To let the air help heal the sores and blisters, wear loose-fitting cotton underwear. Then try any of the following tips:

Break off a leaf from the aloe vera plant, squeeze out the gel, and apply it directly on the sores.

Or, squeeze out the oil from a vitamin E capsule and put it on the sores. We were told that if you use the oil the second you feel the symptoms coming on, it may actually prevent them from blossoming.

Arginine, an amino acid, is said to promote the growth of this nasty virus. Eliminate foods that are rich in arginine: chocolate, peas, chicken soup, veal, lamb, beef, bran, buckwheat, nuts, seeds, gelatin, grain cereals, cola, and beer.

L-lysine, another amino acid, seems to discourage the virus from taking hold. Eat steamed flounder—a half-pound, twice in one day, may rid you of symptoms. Other foods rich in L-lysine are avocado, pumpernickel, lima beans, lentils, potatoes, cottage cheese, and shrimp. You can supplement your diet with L-lysine tablets—500 mgs before lunch and 500 mgs before dinner.

Megadoses of vitamin C have also been proven effective in quickly clearing up herpes symptoms and, in some cases, making them go bye-bye forever.

Take 1,000 mgs of vitamin C every hour, ten hours a day, for ten days. Well, we *did* say "megadoses!" Be consistent with the 10,000 mgs a day for the ten days. If you notice any unpleasant side effects from the vitamin C, stop taking it. Be sure to check with your doctor *before* taking megadoses of *anything!*

Gem Therapy: Choose either sodalite or sugilite. Both stones are said to help release guilt, clear the mind of emotional confusion, and help one get in touch with one's inner strength.

℘ **Affirmation:** Repeat the affirmation at least ten times, first thing in the morning, last thing at night, and throughout the day, right after you have a lustful thought. (It may happen more often than you realize, so be prepared to say the affirmation a whole lot.)

I am a special person. Part of my specialness is my sexuality. My body gives me pleasure without guilt.

REFERRALS

For free information, a confidential consultation, and treatment referral, all paid for by the federal government, call:

Sexually Transmitted Disease Hotline
8 A.M.–11 P.M. E.S.T.—Mon–Fri
800/227-8922

National Herpes Hotline
9 A.M.–7 P.M. E.S.T.
919/361-8488

HICCUPS

Hiccups are a spasm of the diaphragm. The *hic* sound is caused by air being sucked in, then stopped short by tightened vocal cords. It's the least serious ailment, for which we have the most remedies.

You all know the classics: Drink sugar and water or take a teaspoon of sugar; hold your breath (Joany's favorite is to hold her breath and think of ten bald men); drink water from the far side of the glass; place a piece of silverware in a glass of water and drink the water with the handle of the silverware against your temple; place a handkerchief over a glass of water and sip the water through the hanky; and the ol' index fingers in your ears while someone holds a glass of water for you to drink.

Here are some soon-to-be classic remedies to amuse you, to amaze you, and to make you look forward to your next case of hiccups.

• Hold a penny between any two toes of one foot and transfer the penny to any two toes of the other foot, being careful not to let it touch the floor.

• Have a calcium fix. Mash a piece of chalk the width of the average pinky nail and eat it.

• Stand on your head for a couple of minutes.

• Follow your pinkies straight down to the end of your palm till you come to those last tufts. Use those tufts to gently press on your eyeballs for no more than a minute.

• Try aromatherapy. Take long, deep whiffs of sandalwood oil.

- Care for a spot of tea? The verdict is in. Dill seed tea is the most effective tea for hiccups. Use one teaspoon of dill seeds in a cup of just-boiled water. Don't *dilly-*dally—strain and drink as soon as it's cool enough.

- A favorite among bartenders is a wedge of lemon with Worcestershire sauce sprinkled on it. Billy Tull, NBC Property Master, recommends Angostura bitters on lemon.

- Try the ice cure—some say place an ice bag right below the rib cage; others say the ice bag should go on the pit of the stomach. Wherever, keep it there for three to five minutes.

- Light a match and blow it out, then dip the burned portion in a half glass of water and drink the water. The combination of *blowing* and *drinking* should rid you of the hiccups.

- Remember the old hiccup remedy where you breathe in a brown paper bag a few times? We have an update on it, with specific instructions that make it a sure cure.
  Scrunch the neck of a brown paper bag and form a circle around your mouth, allowing no air to escape. Now, taking short, strong, hard breaths, inhale and exhale ten times—no more, no less. When you're finished, don't be surprised if your face is flushed. Do be surprised if you still have the hiccups.

- As a last resort, massage your feet for five to ten minutes. The middle of the bottoms of your feet, right below the balls of your feet, are the pressure points for the diaphragm. This deep massage can stop hiccups if everything else fails.
  Or, take a cotton swab and, for a minute, carefully massage the soft section in back of the roof of your mouth.

Hiccup Prevention: It is said that if you wear a nutmeg around your neck, you will not get the hiccups. But then again, think of all the fun you'd be missing by not trying out some of these remedies.

When Someone Else Has the Hiccups: Suddenly, accuse that person of something of which they are not guilty: *"You*

forgot to give me a message!'' ''What a mess you made in the other room!''
''You better stop spreading those rumors!''

Or, give the hiccupper a penny without telling them why.
The hiccups should stop instantly, as long as they take and hold
that penny.

Since "Home is where the heart is," you've got to protect your heart along with your other organs by making sure your home is well-ventilated and as pollution-free as possible. These suggestions can help—

NATURAL AIR POLLUTION FIGHTERS

After extensive research conducted by the National Aeronautics and Space Administration (NASA), it was concluded that specific common house plants can dramatically reduce toxic chemical levels in homes and offices.

If you're thinking to yourself that your home isn't polluted—after all, you open the bathroom window when you use that tile spray—take a look at this list of common toxins lurking in your living quarters: benzene (found in inks, oils, paints, plastics, rubber, detergents, dyes, and gasoline); formaldehyde (found in all indoor environments, including foam insulation, particle board, pressed wood products, most cleaning agents, paper products treated with resins, including grocery bags, facial tissues, and paper towels); and trichloroethylene (TCE, which is found in dry-cleaning processes, printing inks, paints, lacquers, varnishes, and adhesives).

We will spare you the details on the serious harm these chemicals can do. Instead, here's a list of plants that proved effective in reducing the levels of the common toxins:

• Spider Plant (chlorophytum comosum "vittatum")—very easy to grow in indirect or bright-diffused light.

• Peace Lily (spathiphyllum species)—very easy to grow in low light location.

- Chinese Evergreen (aglaonema "silver queen")—very easy to grow in low light location.

- Weeping Fig (ficus benjamina)—easy to grow, but requires a little special attention. Needs indirect or bright-diffused light.

- Golden Pothos (epipremnum aureum)—very easy to grow in indirect or bright-diffused light.

NASA recommends placing fifteen to eighteen of these plants in an 1,800 square-foot home to clean and refresh the air. Most of us living in apartments or houses with much less space need just a plant in each room. Place plants where air circulates.

And, once you have the plants, don't be surprised if you or members of your household don't complain any more of sore throats and stuffy noses that were caused by contaminants.

Home-grown Love: A little less scientific than the NASA information above, but a lot more romantic, is the notion that sprouting an avocado pit will spread love throughout your home. Why? Because the avocado is ruled by Venus—and because we say so!

Dusting Tip: Before you take out a vacuum cleaner, use a damp cloth to dust. The vacuum's exhaust blows the dust from one place to another.

For Ant- and Worm-Free Wood: Squeeze out the gel from the leaves of an aloe vera plant and use it as a varnish on the woodwork and wood furniture in your home, to protect the wood from worms and white ants.

Stained Glass Light: Stained glass windows, lamps, and chandeliers refract light and create rainbows that add to the positive flow of energy in the house.

Fireplace Alert: Do not feed the fire in your fireplace with colored magazines and colored newspapers. They contain lead and when burned they emit dangerous levels of lead. It can be extremely harmful, especially to children in the house.

Oven Cleaning: Phyllis Diller, not known for her talent as a housekeeper, got a big laugh with, "There is such a buildup of crud in my oven, there's only room to bake a single cupcake!"

If, unlike Ms. Diller, you clean your oven and if you use a commercial oven cleaner, especially one that has non-methane hydrocarbons, open all your windows. If you have an exhaust fan, turn it on "high"—the fumes from the cleaner can be harmful. Stay out of harm's way. Don't go into your kitchen for a few hours. Better yet, leave your house for a while.

Once the oven is clean, you can get rid of the awful smell of the cleaner in your oven by baking orange peels at 350°F.

Trash Compactor Deodorizer: Three to five drops of oil of wintergreen in your trash compactor will make it tolerable until it's emptied.

Home Sweet-Smelling Home: Boil a few cinnamon sticks in a quart of water. By the time the water is almost boiled away, your whole house will be bathed in the lovely scent of cinnamon.

Healing Color: Artist and color authority Laurie Zagon explains that *color* and *light* are the same thing. It was proven when Sir Isaac Newton created the seven spectrum colors by passing a beam of light through a prism.

Light heals; people feel better in the light; the more light, the greater sense of security and optimism. According to Laurie, you can create the essence of light through the seven spectrum colors of the rainbow: red, orange, yellow, green, blue, indigo, and violet, and thus create a healing environment.

If you feel that painting your room with the seven pure colors would be too overpowering, add white to the colors for a pastel version of the rainbow. You might want to accessorize the room with flowers, a bedspread, draperies, and wall hangings in the pure spectrum colors.

INDIGESTION

The typical American consumes about a ton of food and drink annually. *That's two thousand pounds a year!* No wonder we have indigestion.

Here are remedies to remedy that awful feeling—

• Take tea and see . . . see how fast any one of the following can settle your stomach: peppermint tea, camomile, raspberry, sage, fennel, caraway, anise, dill, parsley, and blackberry, all available at health food stores. If you buy yours loose rather than in tea bags, use a heaping teaspoon in a cup of just-boiled water. Let it steep seven to ten minutes, strain, and drink . . . slowly.

• Potatoes can neutralize the acid that may be causing indigestion. Peel and grate a potato, then strain it through cheesecloth, collecting the juice. Add an equal amount of water and drink it slowly for fast relief.

• Papaya, pineapple, mango, and kiwi all have healing enzymes. If you can get the fresh ripe fruit, eat a portion as dessert.

If the fruit isn't available, drink papaya and/or pineapple juice. Make sure the juice is additive-free.

If you don't have juice, take four papaya pills after a meal. The fruit, juice, and pills are the best-tasting medicine around.

• Grate the peel of a grapefruit. Spread out the tiny grated crumbs to dry on paper towels. Then put them in a jar with a lid, label it, and put it in your medicine cabinet (it keeps quite a while). Whenever you have an upset stomach, take up to a teaspoon of the grapefruit crumbs. Chew them, making sure you saturate them with your saliva. Good-bye Tums. Hello crumbs!

• Ah, the glamour of show business . . . traveling to exotic places to shoot a film . . . eating the traditional food of the area. California producer Jill Alman shared her on location/upset stomach remedy with us. It's the BRAT diet. For two or three days she eats only *B*ananas, *R*ice, *A*pples, and *T*oast.

Reflexology: Vigorously massage the instep of each foot. Start in the center, right below the ball of the foot, and work your way toward the outer edge. There should be a particularly sensitive spot on each foot. Those spots correspond directly with the stomach. Once you've found them, dig in with your thumb and knuckles as you continue the deep massage for seven minutes or more, if you have the stamina to continue.

Gem Therapy: Peridot is a yellow-green stone that, according to Joyce and Connie, proprietors of the gem shop Crystal Gardens, helps release emotional tension when placed on the solar plexus (the pit of the stomach). That emotional tension can be the cause of indigestion and the stone can help be the cure.

Another stone suggested by the gemologists is citrine. It's golden in color and good for cleansing the digestive system.

Color Therapy: The color "yellow" emits energy that helps heal inside the belly. Wear yellow clothing; sleep on a yellow sheet; write on yellow legal pads; have yellow flowers near you; and tie a yellow ribbon 'round—anything in view. It's easy to remember this remedy. Just think of "yellow belly."

Prevention: Yes, you can have your cake and eat it too. It's even possible to have a whole holiday meal and not regret it, if you have an indigestion-prevention cocktail first.

Mix one tablespoon of honey and one tablespoon of apple cider vinegar in a cup of warm water. Drink it at least fifteen minutes before you sit down to eat. Happy holiday!

🎵 **Affirmation:** At the first sign of indigestion, relax and repeat at least a dozen times—

I let go of my fears and I am left with my gifts. I am now willing to share my gifts with the world, and the world is willing to accept them.

GAS

A senior citizen neighbor keeps telling us, "When I was young, life was a gas. Now, gas is my life!"

Gas seems to be a problem at any age. For the most part, gas is caused by air that's swallowed when you eat—especially if you eat fast. Loose-fitting dentures can cause intestinal gas; so does drinking through a straw, drinking carbonated beverages, sucking on candy, chewing gum, smoking, and constipation.

There are certain foods and combinations of foods that cause gas. Chances are you know which foods affect you in this way. The remedy for that is simple . . . stay away from those foods.

Here are some more simple remedies to help relieve this uncomfortable condition—

• Cut three or four quarter-size slices of fresh ginger root and drop them in a big mug of just-boiled water. Let it steep for ten minutes. Strain and drink right after a gas-causing meal or any time you have gas pains.

• Take a tablespoon of aloe vera gel after every meal or whenever you feel trapped air bubbles in your stomach.

• Do a headstand (if you are used to doing a headstand). Stay upside down for just a minute. This temporary, drastic position change can help relieve blocked gas.

• Pantothenic acid (vitamin B-5) is reputed to help maintain a healthy digestive tract. A daily dose of 250 mgs has also been known to clear up cases of gastritis.

• After eating, drink a cup of any one of the following herb teas: peppermint, camomile, yarrow, or sage.

• After a gas-producing meal, a cup of any one of the following herb seed teas can help prevent gas buildup: anise, fenugreek, caraway, fennel, or dill seeds. Crush a teaspoon of the seeds and put them in a cup of just-boiled water. Let it steep for ten minutes. Strain and drink.

• The enzymes in papaya pills can help you digest food and eliminate gas. Chew four of the candylike pills after every meal.

They're perfect to carry with you when you eat out, so don't leave home without 'em.

• Drink an ounce of warm, pure virgin olive oil and take a walk, but not too far from a bathroom.

• When you're cooking beans, throw in a few pieces of potatoes. When the beans are ready, take out the potato pieces and the gas should go out with them.

If you do eat beans that weren't prepared properly, eat a piece of watermelon right after the beans, and you'll have fewer repercussions.

Acupressure: Massage the insteps of the bottom of your feet for about ten minutes. It should help release trapped gas.

Aromatherapy: At the first sign of a gas pain, put a couple of drops of essential geranium oil on your wrist and take a few deep whiffs.

Prevention: Put a half-level-teaspoon of yellow mustard seeds in a half-cup of water and drink it down without chewing the seeds. Do this a half hour before lunch and a half hour before dinner. It can make a tremendous difference.

♪ **Affirmation:** At the first sign of a gas pain, or a bloated feeling, relax and repeat at least a dozen times—
I let confidence push fears out of my body and I am blessed with well-being.

HEARTBURN

Heartburn is not a burn and does not affect the heart. It's an irritation caused by too much acid backing up from the stomach to the esophagus. That's what it should be called, "acid backup." Somehow that just doesn't have a ring to it.

Whatever you call it, it's unpleasant and is usually caused by smoking, having caffeine (that means coffee, nonherbal tea, chocolate, aspirin, or cola), eating animal fats, fried and spicy foods, tomato products and other acid-producing food, falling asleep soon after you've eaten, and, another major factor, stress—known in my family as "aggravation."

When you think of all the things you do, have, and eat that can cause heartburn, isn't it amazing that you don't get it more often?

Here are some remedies for when you do have the discomfort of heartburn—

• Slippery elm bark (available at health food stores) neutralizes acid, absorbs gas, and helps digestion too. Use one level teaspoon of slippery elm powder, or one heaping teaspoon of slippery elm bark, in a cup of just-boiled water. Drink it slowly. It can make a big difference in a little amount of time.

• Mix two tablespoons of pure virgin olive oil with an egg white. Don't think about it, just drink it down.

• Take a pinch of coffee grounds, let your saliva mix with them for a minute or two, and spit them out.

We would think it *causes* heartburn rather than cures it, but the woman who gave us the remedy told us to try it. Actually, we had friends try it (our mother didn't raise stupid children), and they said it works.

• Put two iceberg lettuce leaves (about four ounces) along with six ounces of cold water in a blender and push "purée." Pour the thickish greenish liquid into a glass, and drink slowly.

Prevention: Do not lie down right after you've eaten. In fact, wait two to three hours before you assume a prone position, or be prepared to assume the risk of heartburn.

Chronic heartburn sufferers might consider raising the head of the bed by placing six-inch blocks under the legs. Be sure it's done by a carpenter or someone who knows how to properly secure the blocks in place.

NAUSEA

In order to deal most effectively with nausea, you should figure out the reason for it.

Are you "sick to your stomach" about some situation or relationship in your life? If that's why you're feeling awful, then confront whatever it is and work it out. A good cry may also relieve tension and the nausea.

Are you taking any medication? It can cause nausea. Check with your doctor.

If you're nauseous because you've had too much alcohol, you're in the wrong section of the book. You want "Hangover" under ALCOHOLISM AND SOCIAL DRINKING.

Are you pregnant? Check "Morning Sickness" under PREGNANCY.

Are you feeling nauseous in a plane, train, or car? Turn to the chapter on MOTION SICKNESS.

Did you overeat or eat foods that didn't agree with you? This is the place!

NAUSEA REMEDIES

• The classic remedy for nausea is ginger ale. Sip it slowly. Or, even more effective is to dissolve a half-teaspoon of ginger powder in a cup of warm water and drink it down. If you prefer the real thing, take four quarter-size slices of ginger root and steep them for ten minutes in a cup of just-boiled water. Strain and drink.

• A strong cup of peppermint tea is calming to the system and settling to the stomach.

If you have fresh peppermint leaves, crush them and put them on your stomach, touching your bare skin, of course. Bind them in place and stay seated, rather than lying down.

• You may want to eat a bowl of barley. It's a soothing food particularly effective for digestive disorders that cause nauseousness.

• This is a traditional New England remedy that requires a large nutmeg. Using a nutmeg grater, grate it down to half its size. Flat side up, put it under the broiler until oil seeps out of it. As soon as the broiled nutmeg is cool enough to touch, tape it, flat side down, to the pit of your stomach. Once all the heat has gone out of it, reheat it and put it back in place.

- If you can eat something, make it half of a peeled cucumber. It should have a calming, cooling effect on your digestive system.

At a Hotel: If you don't want to get more nauseous when you get the room service bill for a bottle of ginger ale, then get a free bucket of ice from the ice machine in the hall. Chewing on ice chips can cure nauseousness.

When You're Outdoors: There you are, outside, not near a kitchen or a restaurant, and you feel nauseous. What should you do? Pick up a newspaper—make sure it's black and white—and sniff the ink. Yes, you read that correctly. We've gotten forms of this remedy from many people. One woman who wrote to us said that it works every time, even when she has a mild stomach virus. It doesn't cure the virus; it just instantly eliminates the nauseousness.

Reflexology: Dig your thumbs into the area between the second and third toes of each foot and massage deeply for at least five minutes. Rest, then start again. If, after ten minutes of massage, you no longer feel nauseous, it worked.

✒ **Affirmation:** At the first wave of nausea, relax and repeat over and over—
   I am free of fear. I now know that I am in the right place, at the right time, and I am doing the right thing.

STOMACH RUMBLING

Those embarrassing rumbling sounds that are loudest during a job interview and at what otherwise would have been a romantic moment are caused by intestinal wall contractions and the movement of gas and liquid.

If you're playing Trivial Pursuit and you're asked for the medical term for the rumbling sounds, the answer is "borborygmus."

If you're asked what to do to prevent it, here are some suggestions. The first is this: Instead of having three meals a day, have more than three but eat a lot less at each meal. The second: Cut down on the amount of air you swallow. That means:

• Don't gulp down food. Eat slowly.

• Don't drink very hot beverages. They cause you to swallow air in an attempt to cool the drink.

• When you drink, keep your upper lip in the liquid. That way, air won't be gulped down or sipped in.

• Avoid aerated foods—things that are put through a blender or whipped in some way.

• If all these rules make you sigh, don't! Sighing also causes you to swallow air.

For Special Occasions: When you're on television with a microphone in your lapel, you don't want your stomach to go into competition with you. TV producer Nahmee Han said that a show biz remedy to prevent stomach rumbling is to eat a banana right before "show time." It works for us!

INFANTS—
NEWBORN TO AGE TWO

The ovaries of every human female at birth contain two million eggs—give or take a few. Only about 300,000 eggs survive to puberty and, during a woman's reproductive years, about 450 are released for possible fertilization.

The human male's testes manufacture 15 billion sperm cells each month, and 400 million sperm are released in a single ejaculation.

This means that 1 out of 450 eggs merged with 1 sperm out of 400 million to form a single-celled zygote. That single cell miraculously divided into more than 100 trillion cells to become a very special human being—*your* baby.

Cuddle, cradle, caress, hold, hug, and love your baby! Studies show that babies who are hugged and loved are healthier, grow faster, cry less, and are more active.

We know you know this, but we couldn't sleep nights if we didn't say it anyway: *Check with your pediatrician before trying any of the following remedies on your baby.*

Air Travel: In an airplane, takeoff and landing can be particularly painful to baby's sensitive little ears. To help make the flight as comfortable as possible, especially during takeoff and landing, feed your baby a bottle of whatever (s)he prefers to drink. The constant swallowing can help equalize ear pressure.

Colds/Chest Congestion: In a pan, combine one slice of white bread with a quarter-cup of milk and a pinch of catnip. Heat it for a minute or two. Then put it in a white cotton sock. Make sure it's cool enough to put on the baby's chest to help clear up the congestion and the cold.

Colic: There are dozens of reasons and any number of combinations of reasons that can cause colic. There are also many treatments or combinations of treatments for it. Use that inner voice to help you decide which would work best for your baby.

• If you are nursing, you may be feeding the baby too often, not allowing enough time for proper digestion. Try for longer intervals between nursing sessions and see if that makes a difference.

• If baby is on cow's milk, add a teaspoon of acidophilus (available at health food stores) to the bottle. Make sure the label says there are one to two billion viable acidophilus cells.

• This wins the contest for the most unique remedy: Set your baby on the top of a clothes dryer that's in use. *Stand in front of the dryer, making sure baby is safe. Do not walk away or even turn away for one second!*
Or, put the baby, in its infant seat, against the side of a clothes dryer that's doing a load.
In either case the heat, the vibration, and the hum seems to comfort a colicky child.

• When you're finished with the laundry (above), you may want to vacuum. Good. The noise of a vacuum cleaner may calm the colic baby, especially if you vacuum while carrying your child in a front carrier. Even if your baby doesn't stop fussing, at least you'll have a clean home.

• Put a small slice of onion in a half-cup of water and let it boil for a minute. Then add a quarter-teaspoon of sugar and let it cool. Take out the onion and give the sugared onion water to the baby. Within a half hour the colic should be gone.

• Turn your radio to a station that's not broadcasting but still has the dead air sound called *white noise.* That no-sound sound has been known to calm some colicky kids.

• Dill seed tea can relieve colic and prevent it from recurring. Prepare the dill seed (available at health food stores) by steeping a half-teaspoon in a covered cup of just-boiled water for six minutes. Stir, then strain. When it's cool enough, give the baby two to four ounces of the dill tea.

- In the morning, an hour before the first feeding, give baby a teaspoon of olive oil. We've heard that this works fast. Within a few days colic may be history.

Cradle Cap: Puncture a vitamin E capsule, squeeze out the oil, and gently massage it on the baby's scaley scalp. If one application doesn't clear up the condition, repeat the treatment the next day.

Diaper Rash: There are harmless bacteria that live on skin and feed on urea, the nitrogen part of urine. Their waste product is ammonia, which causes diaper rash.

These bacteria are anaerobic. That means that oxygen kills them. When babies are bundled up with a diaper and plastic pants, air can't get in and so the bacteria thrive, producing ammonia, which causes diaper rash. The answer is to let air get at the baby's skin. That means, lose the plastic covering! Treat a severe case of diaper rash by letting the baby romp around bare-bottom as much as possible, until the condition clears up.

There's an old folk remedy for diaper rash, and if it worked way back when, there's no reason it shouldn't work now. Pour three cups of flour in a heavy fry pan, over a medium-to-high flame. Stir it with a wooden spoon until it turns a darkish brown, without burning. Bottle it and use it in place of talcum powder every time you change baby's diaper.

If you don't have flour for the remedy above, and you do have corn starch, put corn starch on the diaper. It can help make baby more comfortable and clear up the rash, too.

Diarrhea: Lots of classic folk remedies require that an ingredient be placed on the soles of the feet. Since the pores on the bottom of a baby's feet are four times larger than anywhere else on the body, you can see how fast-acting an appropriate application might be.

One remedy is to smear the soles of baby's feet with white vinegar. If the condition isn't cleared up in a couple of hours, smear the soles one more time.

Carob has also been used for ages to fight bouts of diarrhea—in adults as well as children. Add one teaspoon of carob powder to baby's water bottle or to apple sauce. Carob is sweet and baby will like it. If diarrhea doesn't stop right away, continue the treatment throughout the day. Don't overdo it. Too much carob can cause constipation!

Finally, you might add a half-teaspoon of fresh lime juice to two ounces of warm water, and if the baby will drink it, the diarrhea may quickly disappear.

Hiccups: Take a little piece of red thread—must be red—and wad it up in your mouth. Put the wadded red thread on your baby's forehead and the hiccups will stop.

Have we ever lied to you?

Gem Therapy for Hiccups: To stop the baby's hiccups, put a piece of rhodochrosite (available at gem stores or see RESOURCES for a mail order contact) on baby's tummy.

Honey—a No-No: Do not give honey to children under one year old. The spores in honey can cause botulism.

Low-Fat Diets: Children who are under two years old should not be on a low-fat diet, even when it comes to milk. In other words, skim milk or low-fat milk should not be fed to your baby or toddler. A fat-restricted diet can lower their defenses against gastrointestinal infections and hamper normal growth and development.

Teething: *Cold* numbs baby's painful, swollen little gums. Let the baby chew on a frozen bagel. The bagel lasts longer than a mushy teething biscuit and can help relieve the pain.

Teething Misconception: Teething does not cause a fever. If your baby is running a fever higher than 101°, chances are the baby is sick, not just teething.

INSECT
STINGS, BITES,
AND REPELLENTS

REMEDIES FOR BEE AND
YELLOW JACKET STINGS AND FLY BITES

If the stinger remains in your skin, do not pull it out with tweezers. The tweezers will squeeze the venom out of the stinger and into you. Just flick the stinger off with your fingers, or scrape it off with a knife.

Chances are, you'll be stung outdoors. Treat the sting with whatever is available. Here are some suggestions:

• Pack mud on the sting.

• Slit open a cigarette, moisten the tobacco, and pack it on the sting.

• Apply your own urine.

• Take a tablespoon of baking soda, add water to make a paste, and put it on the sting.

• Bet you already know about the healing properties of meat tenderizer and water on a sting? Well, you do now.

• Rub on apple cider vinegar.

• Put a slice of raw onion or a peeled, sliced clove of garlic on the sting, wrap a bandage around it, and leave it there for at least two hours.

• Several drops of any one of the following oils—castor oil, cinnamon oil, vitamin E oil, or wheat germ oil—placed on a cotton ball and applied directly on the sting should stop the pain and hold down the swelling.

• If it's already swollen, put an ice pack on it.

SNAKEBITES

A snakebite is serious stuff that, hopefully, will never come up for you. But, if you go camping in deserted, snake-infested areas, you should know about charcoal and *always* carry it with you, just in case you lose your snakebite kit.

If you're bitten by a snake, get to a doctor *immediately!* Until you get professional medical attention, begin treatment quickly, before swelling begins. Open several charcoal capsules, collect the contents, and add enough water to make the consistency of a smooth paste. Apply it directly on the bite, then spread the rest around that area of your skin. Also, as soon as that's done, swallow ten charcoal tablets.

Keep track of the time. Ten minutes after the first application of charcoal powder, scrape it off and put on another layer of the moistened charcoal powder.

The charcoal powder on the bite should draw out and absorb the snake's venom. If the venom gets into your system, the charcoal tablets can absorb it in the gastrointestinal tract.

If the bitten area starts to swell and the pain increases, apply an ice pack (if possible) and continue to take the charcoal pills until you get professional medical help.

MOSQUITO AND HOUSE FLY REPELLENTS

The following repellents are divided into two categories— what you can do to keep mosquitoes away from you, and what you can do to keep mosquitoes away from your home—

• Garlic—eat lots of raw garlic, take garlic pills, and/or rub garlic on your exposed areas.

• Onions—eat a raw onion or two daily and a mosquito won't dare come near you.

• Parsley—rub sprigs of it on your exposed areas.

• Apple cider vinegar—rub it or spray it on your exposed skin.

• Be sugar-free and alcohol-free and you'll be mosquito-free.

• Brewer's yeast—take two tablespoons daily with your meals to prevent being mosquitoes' meals.

- The smell of citronella is known to repel insects. You can sprinkle the essential oil concentrate (available at herb shops and some health food stores) where needed. Other oils that are as effective are eucalyptus, rosemary, and pennyroyal.

- Hang bouquets of dried tomato leaves in each room to repel mosquitoes. This works for flies and spiders as well.

- In Europe, window boxes abound. They not only look pretty, they keep house flies away. You can, too, by having any of these easy-to-grow insect-repelling plants on your window ledges, near doorways, and on patios or terraces: sweet basil, tansy, fennel, bay.

Mosquito Bite Itch Prevention: You have about 3 minutes after you've been bitten to neutralize the element in the mosquito's saliva that causes the itch. Quick!—reach for the baking soda. Pour a little in your palm and make a paste of it by adding some water. Then smear it on the bite. Time's up! You're still looking for the baking soda? Put it where it's handy when needed.

Gnat Repellent: If you're going into a gnat-infested area, protect yourself by coating your exposed body parts with a thin layer of baby oil.

Ant Repellents: If you have an ant problem, do a thorough clean-up job of the area(s) they frequent, then use one or more of these *ant*idotes—

- Dried bay leaves—good for kitchen cabinets—they lose their effectiveness after about a year.

- Coffee grounds—good for doors and windows.

- Petroleum jelly—fill in the cracks in walls or around the sink.

- Mint leaves—plant them near entrances and windows and terraces.

- Cayenne pepper—good in cabinets or on counter tops.

- Fresh lemon juice—with a medicine dropper, drip the juice in floorboard cracks, window sills, and door jambs.

- Whole cloves—wedge them into corners of cabinets, drawers, or wherever the ants are entering your home.

Yellow Jacket Repellent: When you're having a picnic outdoors and don't want any univited guests flying in to join you, pour apple cider vinegar in a couple of saucers and place them around your picnic area.

Lyme Tick Repellent: Chrysanthemums attract Lyme ticks and have a substance that then kills them. This is interesting information that, unfortunately, won't help when you're romping in the park. In other words, even if you're holding a bouquet of chrysanthemums, you still have to tuck your pants into your socks for protection against those little buggers.

Moth Repellents: When you're ready to store your winter woolens, go to an herb shop for either dried lavender, pennyroyal leaves, or cedar chips. They will repel moths as effectively as camphor mothballs, but with a much more pleasant fragrance.

Dry-Food Worms Repellent: When dry food like cereals, beans, and flour are stored in your kitchen cupboards for a while, particularly in warm weather, you may find some added protein in there that you didn't pay for . . . and don't want. Prevent worms, grain beetles, and other creepy-crawlies from invading your vittles by putting a couple of dried bay leaves in each box or sack of dry food.

REFERRAL

For more information on pesticides and the safe way to get rid of insects, write to or call:

National Coalition Against the Misuse of Pesticides
701 E Street S.E. Suite 200
Washington, DC 2003
202/543-5450

ITCHING

What can cause skin to itch? Dryness, heat, allergies, certain lotions, ointments, creams, and medications that end with "-dryl" or "-caine."

Try not to scratch an itch (that's easy for us to say!), since scratching can cause infection. And give an itchy patch a few days to clear up. If it stays red, raw, or oozes, and if it gets worse with treatment rather than better, get professional medical help.

• Dip a white washcloth in milk, wring it out, and place the wet cloth on the itchy area.

• Moisten the itchy area with water. Then take a pinch of salt (coarse kosher salt is preferable) and rub it on that same area. Stop when the itching stops—probably in a few minutes.

• Eat foods that are rich in iron—green leafy vegetables, fish, dried fruits, wheat germ, and cherry juice.

• Do not wear loud, bright, hot colors like red, shocking pink, fuchsia, or orange. They seem to encourage itching. Blue, on the other hand (or on any other part of your body), can actually help stop the itching.

Possible Causes of Rectal Itching: Cut down considerably on caffeine, or cut it out completely. That means coffee, cola, and chocolate. If, within two days, the itching stops, chances are you have a sensitivity to caffeine and through trial and error—make that, trial and itching—you'll discover the amount of caffeine your body will tolerate.

Tomatoes, citrus juices, and beer can also cause rectal itching. It's easy enough to find out. Just eliminate the suspected food or drink from your diet for two or three days. If the itching stops . . . bingo!

A common cause of rectal itching is yeast overgrowth. Go on a yeast-free diet and watch for results.

Rectal Itch Remedies: Instead of soap, use apple cider vinegar to wash the rectal area.

Or, spread plain yogurt on a sanitary napkin and place it on the itchy area. Change the dressing every couple of hours.

Jock Itch: This fungal infection of the groin is contagious. Don't scratch it—you can spread it to other parts of your body including your scalp (it's then called "ringworm").

Three times a day, apply the oil from garlic capsules to the parasitic patches until it clears up completely.

To eliminate the ideal conditions for growing fungus, wear loose-fitting, cotton underwear to keep air in and moisture out.

KOMBUCHA TEA MUSHROOM

In January of 1995, we were on the "Maury Povich Show," and included the Kombucha Tea Mushroom in our segment, since it was the newest oldest remedy we had.

With a limited amount of TV time to devote to the Kombucha, we demonstrated and explained: the Mushroom-growing process begins with the preparation of a distilled water-sugar-tea in a stainless steel pot which is then replaced by a glass bowl. When it has cooled to room temperature, you float the Kombucha Tea Mushroom (which you bought or were given) in the bowl, add the starter tea that comes with the Kombucha, cover it, and put it in a quiet, dark, clean place for 7 to 10 days. At the end of that time, you take out the bowl, uncover it, and—if all went well—you will see that the Kombucha has cloned itself. The original Kombucha has become a *mom* and the *baby* is attached to it. You peel the *mom* and the *baby* apart, replant (or refloat) the *mom* in a newly-prepared brew and either do the same with the *baby,* or give it away. Then, strain into a glass bottle the liquid that the Kombuchas were in, and refrigerate what is now your health tonic.

We talked about the Kombucha for about five minutes on the "Maury Povich Show," and that was enough time to totally confuse and titillate the TV viewers. The day the show aired, and for days afterward, records were set for the number of phone calls received by the Povich production office, as well as at our publisher's toll-free order number. And our post office box was bursting at the seams with letters asking about the "Kombotcha," "Choobooky," "Bahkoochy," "Shamboola," "You know, that mushroom thing."

The Kombucha (pronounced: Calm *boo* shaa) is not a mushroom. Okay, so if the Kombucha Tea Mushroom is *not* a mushroom, then what is it . . . other than strange, fascinating and health-giving?

Betsy Pryor, President of Laurel Farms, who introduced the Kombucha to the American public in 1993, calls it "a gift from God."

It's also one of the reasons for this book's revision . . . to introduce this intriguing phenomenon to you, to answer any questions you may have about the Kombucha Tea Mushroom, and to give you enough information to help you decide whether this ongoing process is something you want for your health.

Your first question might be, *What in the world is it and where did it come from?* Betsy Pryor answered this for us. "Even though it's called a Kombucha Tea Mushroom or a Manchurian Mushroom or a Kargasok Mushroom, or any of the dozens of other names it's acquired in the past several thousand years, the Kombucha isn't *really* a mushroom at all. In fact, the Kombucha doesn't exist in nature. *Someone* put it together. Just who, remains a mystery.

"Although it's widely believed that the Kombucha existed as early as 220 B.C. in China where it was known as the Divine Tea, I believe that its origins go back much farther in time, perhaps 4,500 years. I have a *hunch* (I'm an amateur Egyptologist) that the *someone* was an Egyptian, someone skilled in the fine Egyptian art of fermentation, perhaps a healer living in the time of the Pharaoh Khufu, the builder of the Great Pyramid, and that it made its way to China via an ancient spice route *later.*

"It's a symbiotic combination of good bacteria and yeast (not the kind that causes yeast problems), that when left alone for 7–10 days floating in a mixture of ordinary sugar, tea, and water, combines to make an invigorating beverage containing vitamins B1, B2, B3, B6, B12, folic acid, and glucuronic acid, which works with the liver to bind up environmental and metabolic toxins and excrete them from the body. Glucuronic acid is also a precursor of a group of important mucopolysaccharides, the building blocks of the human body.

"The Kombucha also makes a new *baby* that can be kept or given away. Legend has it that the babies of your original *mom* Kombucha will, if treated kindly, accompany you for life."

Why would I want to even consider using this? Good question! The Kombucha "tea" is said to be a super immune booster, assisting the body in fighting everything from yeast infections and ulcers to psoriasis, arthritis, constipation, chronic diarrhea, prostate problems, male and female incontinence, hemorrhoids, stress, chronic fatigue syndrome, indigestion, kidney and gallstones, high cholesterol, acne, diabetes, multiple sclerosis, cancer, raising T-cell counts, hardening of the arteries, memory loss and other symptoms of aging, menopausal symptoms, PMS, impotence, wrinkles, weight problems, gout, carpal tunnel syndrome, hypoglycemia, hair loss, and heaven-only-knows-what-else. People tell us it's great for their pets, too. Putting a few eyedroppersful in their drinking water each day adds sparkle and new life to their skin, coat, and disposition, and can eliminate "doggy breath."

It sounds like a cure-all. Is it? No! We've been involved with the Kombucha since October 1994. While we know people who have accomplished miraculous results by drinking the tea, we also know people who started and stopped because they didn't feel they were receiving enough benefits from the tea to make it worthwhile.

So, how do I know if it will be beneficial for me? The only way is by trying it. That's why we want you to know more about it, and exactly what's involved in the growing and harvesting processes of the Kombucha.

What do I need? What do I do? How do I do it? And when? Before you get the Kombucha Tea Mushroom, you should gather enough supplies to get started:

a 3–4 quart glass mixing bowl
flour sacking towels (white cotton fabric)
4 quart stainless steel pot
green tea bags/black tea bags
a few 6 inch rubber bands
a wooden or plastic spoon
1 cup white (ordinary refined) cane or beet sugar
a gallon of distilled water
measuring pitcher (for quarts of water)
tape (Scotch tape works fine)

Once you have the supplies, you're ready for the Mushroom. Chances are, you already know someone who is *doing* the Kombucha—someone with integrity and clean growing conditions whom you trust—and who will be happy to give you a Mushroom. Or, you can order a Mushroom from a commercial grower. There are growers throughout the country, many of whom sell through health food stores. As you may have guessed, we refer people to Laurel Farms where Betsy Pryor, and her devoted staff, have grown over 10,000 Kombuchas and are still going strong. Betsy has graciously agreed to share their instructions with us.

We've edited Betsy's instructions down to the bare bones, presenting what we hope is a clear picture of this ongoing process. Once you're ready for "hands on," you will, most likely, have the step-by-step instructions that will make it a cinch to successfully prepare, grow, and harvest the Kombucha Tea Mushroom.

When Your Kombucha Arrives: You will probably receive the Kombucha Tea Mushroom in an airtight plastic bag. The first thing you're gonna do is open the airtight plastic bag to let your Kombucha Tea Mushroom breathe. Make sure you don't spill the tea inside, because you're gonna need it to start the fermenting process. Do not let your Kombucha Tea Mushroom come into contact with metal, direct sunlight, or microwaves.

Preparation of the "Growing Tea": Bring 3 quarts of water (distilled or nonchlorinated) to a boil in your stainless steel pot. Add 1 cup sugar and boil for another 5 minutes. Turn off water, add 4 tea bags. Remove after 10 minutes. After 20 minutes, pour tea into the 4-quart glass mixing bowl. Cover with a white cotton cloth and let tea cool to room temperature (it takes a few hours).

Planting the Kombucha Tea Mushroom: Add at least 4 ounces of "newly harvested" tea (from your last batch, or in the case of your first Mushroom, add the liquid from the plastic bag). Gently place your Kombucha on top of cooled "growing tea." Place crossed pieces of tape across the bowl. The tape prevents the white cloth from dipping into the "growing tea."

Cover with a white cloth. Put a rubber band around the cloth and bowl. Place bowl in dim or dark, quiet, temperate (70–90 degrees) spot with adequate airflow.

Harvesting and Replanting: After a week to 10 days, prepare another bowl of "growing tea." Take out the bowl with the Mushroom. Remove the white cloth. Notice that the *mom* Kombucha (the one on the bottom) has given birth to a *baby* (the one on the top). Gently separate the two Mushrooms, and replant the "mom" in the bowl with the "growing tea"—the darker side of the Mushroom floating face down.

You now have a "baby" to either replant (depending on how many people for whom you will be providing the Kombucha tea), or give it away. In which case, you will put the "baby" Mushroom in a plastic bag with at least 4 ounces of "growing tea."

Pour the newly-fermented Kombucha health beverage (the 7–10 day old "growing tea") from the glass bowl (using the white cloth as a strainer) into a clear glass refrigerator container. A funnel is a big help here. Place in the refrigerator. Chill, and it's ready to drink.

As with most instructions, it looks more complex than it actually is. Once you get into it, it becomes routine.

What does the tea taste like? It's a fermented drink whose taste varies—probably depending on weather, phases of the moon, and growing conditions—from zingy and sweetish, to zingy and cider vinegary. Some brews are absolutely delicious; others make us pucker just thinking about it. There seems to be no consistency . . . some batches are simply better than others.

How much should I drink a day? The Russian scientists who did a lot of research on the Kombucha said that 4 ounces 3 times a day seemed like a sensible amount. We suggest that people work their way up to 12 ounces a day. Within weeks, you'll get to know the amount that's best for you.

What else should I know about the Kombucha? You should know all of the precautions to take when handling, growing, harvesting and storing the Kombucha and the tea. For example, never expose the Mushroom to direct sunlight. Never let metal (like your jewelry) touch the Mushroom. Use green and/or black (Orange Pekoe) tea for the brew. Herbal teas diminish the health of the Kombucha. Some herbal teas can even kill it. Never use honey instead of sugar. Honey can kill or cripple some of the Kombucha's healthy bacteria, turning it into an ordinary yeast patty.

We don't want to scare you *away*, we just want to scare you so that you will take responsibility for learning the proper way to grow and harvest the Kombucha.

REFERRAL

If you'd like more information about the Laurel Farms strain of the Kombucha Tea Mushroom, send a self-addressed, stamped envelope to:

Laurel Farms
P.O. Box 7405
Studio City, CA 91614

or call 310-289-4372 for a voice presentation.

For those in need, Laurel Farms offers their Kombucha Tea Mushrooms at their shipping and handling cost. Ask for information about this special program.

Neither of us, nor Laurel Farms, makes any claim regarding the health benefits of the Kombucha Tea Mushroom. Always check with your health care professional who knows your medical history before you embark on any self-help treatment.

Please know that we Wilen sisters do not profit financially from Laurel Farms. What we do profit from is knowing that we are helping get valuable information and Mushrooms to people who want it. Dr. Ray Wunderlich, Jr. is the physician who has reviewed and deemed *safe* the remedies in this book. With regard to the Kombucha Tea Mushroom, Dr. Wunderlich says, "The jury is not in yet for this relatively new (very old) product. Just as one may choke on meat, swell up from shrimp, or develop hives from eating eggs, the consumer of Kombucha would wish to use caution lest any strong, able *food* such as this should prove contaminated, toxic, or allergic to the individual user."

See RECOMMENDED READING for Betsy Pryor's book, *Kombucha Phenomenon*.

MASTITIS

Mastitis is an inflammation of the breast. The two common kinds are: acute mastitis involving bacterial infection, and chronic mastitis with no infection, just tenderness and pain.

This is a condition that you should check out with your health professional. Chances are you will be treated with antibiotics. If you are put on antibiotics, be sure to take acidophilus available at health food stores. (Since antibiotics have no discretion, they destroy the good as well as the bad bacteria; therefore you need acidophilus to replace the beneficial bacteria.) Acidophilus capsules should have one to two billion viable acidophilus cells. Read the label carefully.

Important: Take acidophilus right after you've eaten and at least two hours before or two hours after you take an antibiotic. That way you won't make the antibiotic crazy going after the beneficial bacteria in the acidophilus.

Did you know that garlic is a natural antibiotic? You may want to add raw garlic to your diet and supplement it with high-powered garlic perles. A knowledgeable health food store employee can explain your choices.

HOME REMEDIES FOR MASTITIS

The following remedies have been known to work wonders for many women with mastitis.

•   As soon as you feel soreness in your breast, drink violet leaf tea (available at health food stores), two to four cups a day. Use a heaping teaspoon of the leaves to a cup of just-boiled water. Let it steep for ten minutes, then strain and drink. If the breast is inflamed, make a poultice out of the leaves and apply it directly to the breast.

- If you have recurrent mastitis, dandelion leaf tea may be the answer once and for all. Have three cups of the tea (available at health food stores) every day. Also, make a poultice of the leaves and put it on your breast once a day for at least twenty minutes. Expect results within a month.

- A naturopath prescribes 250 mgs of vitamin B-6 daily and 400 IU of vitamin E twice a day. Since vitamin B-6 can be toxic, you should *not* take this dosage for more than a couple of weeks. Note: You should check with your doctor before trying any of these self-help treatments. We mean it . . . especially with this remedy.

𝒮 **Affirmation:** Repeat this affirmation ten times, first thing in the morning, each time you comb or brush your hair, and last thing at night—

I accept myself as a healthy and happy woman, blessed with normal and natural bodily functions.

While doing research, we talk to a lot of people and it seems that everyone—regardless of age—feels as though they're losing their memory. We feel it's data overload.

With television, radio, newspapers, magazines, answering machines, fax machines, and computer modems, we have so much coming at us day and night, it's no wonder we walk into a room and can't remember what we went to get.

Some reassuring information: As we get older, we do lose brain cells, but our aging brains make up for cell loss and actually increase brain functions.

For instance, our interpretive talents heighten as wisdom and judgment deepen. In fact, the ability to speak and write improves after age fifty; philosophers don't reach their peak until seventy or eighty.

So, now that we've eliminated *aging* as a reason for memory loss, let's look at three common causes.

• Depression. When you're depressed, you don't pay very much attention to anything, hindering your ability to create and store new memories.

• Alcohol abuse usually results in memory loss.

• Medication. Memory loss can be a side effect of some medications.

If you are having serious memory problems, worrying about it won't help. Consult a doctor as soon as possible. It may be a chemical imbalance that can be easily remedied.

James M. Barrie, the author of *Peter Pan,* described memory as "What God gave us so that we might have roses in December." Read the suggestions in this chapter, follow the ones appropriate for you—and get out the vase for those roses. Note: You must give the following remedies at least a month, more like two, to get noticeable results.

WAYS TO IMPROVE YOUR MEMORY

Eleanor Roosevelt was known to have an exceptionally good memory. How good was it? It was so good, elephants used to consult with *her!*

We were told that when Mrs. Roosevelt was quite on in years, she was asked to what she attributed her great memory. Her answer was three cloves of garlic a day. It's been reported that Mrs. Roosevelt dipped the garlic cloves in either honey or chocolate.

• The easiest way to eat raw garlic is to finely mince it, put it in water or juice, then just drink it down. If you don't chew the little bits, the smell of garlic won't stay on your breath very long.

• Do mental exercises daily. Watch TV game shows and shout out answers before the contestants do. Do crossword puzzles. Do jigsaw puzzles. Take an adult education course every semester. Write your memoirs. Take up painting. Learn to play the harmonica or the recorder. There's no limit to the stimulating and fun mental exercises out there for you. Use your creativity to find them!

• Take ginkgo capsules. They're available at most health food stores.

The ginkgo biloba tree has existed for over 250 million years. It was the first plant to bloom the following spring after the bomb was dropped on Hiroshima. We're talking about a tree whose resistance to the ravages of time, weather, disease, and atomic energy are legendary. These ginkgo trees have found their way to America and can be seen in most areas of the country. There's a ginkgo tree with its lovely fanlike leaves right outside the building we live in. Those leaves have a substance in them that promotes the flow of oxygen and blood to the brain and that can boost mental alertness.

As for the proper dosage for ginkgo capsules, start by following the recommendation on the label. Most suggest you take two or three capsules or tablets with meals. Be consistent. Also, be patient—it can take up to three months to get results. And be prepared—the pills are fairly expensive.

• Breathe in through your mouth, then breathe out through your nostrils. Keep inhaling through the mouth and exhaling through the nostrils for two minutes, five times throughout the day. This breathing exercise is said to help you turn mental malaise into idea-filled days.

• Throughout the day, drink two to three cups of rosemary and/or sage tea (available at health food stores). Prepare it by adding a cup of just-boiled water to a heaping teaspoon of either herb. Let it steep for ten minutes. Strain and drink.

Forget Forgetfulness: The average American spends a full year of his/her life looking for lost objects. Luckily it's spread out over a long period of time, but you can cut down on that amount of time, not to mention the frustration. Write a list of the half-dozen things you misplace most often. Joan's list is: key, eyeglasses, credit cards, change purse, watch, and gloves. Simply take a *pretend* picture every time you put any of the objects down somewhere. Hold one hand over one eye, make a lenslike circle with the other hand, and look through it with the other eye. Blink as though your eye is a camera taking a picture of the object. An hour, a day, or even a week later, when you need that object, you'll be able to picture exactly where it is.

Improving Short-Term Memory: When you have to learn something you'll be needing real soon (short-term memory)—maybe for a test you're taking, or for a meeting you're going to—go over the information in the *morning*. It could be the morning of the test or meeting, or the morning before. The key word here is *morning* for short-term memory.

Improving Long-Term Memory: Your long-term memory powers are at their peak in the afternoon. If you need to learn something you'll have to recall weeks later, study it between noon and five P.M.

Gem Therapy: The stones for improving one's memory are amethyst and amber calcite. Wear or carry either or both with or on you and your memory should improve. If you remember to get the stones and carry them with you, they're working already.

Aromatherapy: Crush caraway seeds, keep them close by, and every once in a while take a whiff. It's said to strengthen the memory. Vary the whiffing with coriander seeds and ground cloves.

Hot flashes, facial flushes, and night sweats are all part of the spectrum of menopausal symptoms. But according to a study done at the University of Alabama at Birmingham Center for Nursing Research, women who are congruent about their purpose in life have an easier time going through menopause. They experience fewer emotional and physical menopausal symptoms. If you're assertive, independent, and authoritative, you can skip these pages and get on with your life's work. The rest of you, read on.

Breathe Away Flashes: Do this breathing exercise and exorcise those flashes. Breathe in to the count of six; breathe out to the count of six. Do this ten times in a row. Do not pause in between breaths.

The Right Stuff: Wear cotton or wool clothing. The natural fibers will provide more ventilation than synthetics, allowing you to cool off faster from the hot flashes.

Instant Reviver: Rush to the refrigerator and open both doors—the refrigerator part and the freezer part—and stand as close to it as possible. If you're in the street, go into the nearest supermarket and hang out over the frozen food section.

Facial Flushes: Suck on an ice cube. It will cool the blood in the area of the neck and the flushing will be gone in a flash.

Night Sweats: Oatstraw tincture (available at most health food stores) can help prevent night sweats, make you more energetic, and it's good for your skin and hair, too. Take twenty drops in water three times a day, after meals.

• We've all heard good things about ginseng. Many herbalists believe that ginseng is only for men. The comparable *female* Chinese medicinal root is dong quai. It is said to have been used in the Orient for thousands of years to rejuvenate female glands.

For minimizing the symptoms of menopause, we sing the praises of *dong quai* . . . the "Dong Quai Serenade."

Dosage varies depending on the extent of one's symptoms. For average menopause problems, take one capsule of dong quai (available at health food stores) three times a day. For more severe problems, increase dosage accordingly but not excessively. To determine the dosage appropriate for you, check with your health professional.

The powdered herb has a celerylike taste. You can open the capsule and sprinkle the contents on salads or in soups or stews.

Do not eat fruit or drink other strong root teas for at least three hours after taking dong quai.

• Suma is an herb that comes in capsule form, is available at health food and vitamin stores, and is said to be a hormone balancer. Follow the recommended dosage on the label.

Gem Therapy: Chrysocolla is the stone for female problems. It symbolizes wholeness and gives one a sense of peace and well-being. Place it over the third eye (on your forehead, between your two eyes) and you will feel a calm that surrounds you.

♪ **Affirmation:** Repeat this affirmation fifteen times a day, first thing in the morning, every time you look in the mirror, and last thing at night—

I welcome this change in my life. I marvel at my body. It's all happening for my greatest good.

Menstruation

A delicate hormonal balance is responsible for regular menstrual cycles. Therefore, physical or emotional upheaval may be responsible for menstrual irregularities. Keep in mind that some menstrual irregularities can be normal, especially during the early teen years and for several years before menopause. Take a look at your age and your physical and emotional states, then take a look at the rest of this chapter for help.

> **Q:** Why does it take five PMS women to change a light bulb?
>
> **A:** Because . . . *just because!!!*

PMS seems most prevalent in women who are in their thirties and forties. The wide variety of physical and emotional symptoms of PMS are thought to be related to the high level of hormones in the second half of the menstrual cycle, when the estrogen level is higher.

Here are some suggestions for overcoming the biochemical causes of those Problematic Monthly Symptoms.

PREMENSTRUAL SYNDROME (PMS)

• Vitamin B-6 can make a big difference when it comes to *that time of month.* Take one B-6 (100 mgs) daily. You might want to raise the dosage to 150 mgs during the week before you get your period.

Important: Do not take more than 200 mgs of vitamin B-6 a day. It can affect your nervous system.

• Dong quai is a medicinal root used in China to revitalize female glands.

Dosage varies depending on the extent of one's symptoms. For average PMS problems, take one capsule of dong quai (available at health food stores) three times a day. For more severe cases, increase dosage accordingly but not excessively.

• If you eliminate caffeine from your diet (that means coffee, chocolate, aspirin, colas, and more), your pre-period symptoms and the during-your-period pains may not be nearly as troublesome.

• Yarrow tea may be the answer to your period problems. Each of us has had occasion to drink it. It's amazing. Before I even finished the entire cup of tea, my cramps were gone. We've actually changed friends' lives with this remedy . . . women who couldn't cope with PMS and others who had to put their lives on hold while they doubled up in pain during the first two days of their period.

Prepare yarrow tea (available at health food stores) by steeping a teaspoon of the herb in a cup of just-boiled water for about seven minutes. Strain and drink when needed.

MENSTRUAL CRAMPS PREVENTION

• If you have cramps, what should you take? Cramp bark, of course, a Native American remedy. In fact, cramp bark (available at herb shops and some health food stores) is also called squaw bush.

To prevent cramps, drink two cups of cramp bark tea daily, starting a week before you're expecting your period.

Prepare the ground-up cramp bark the way you would the yarrow tea (see above).

• A daily dose of vitamin E (400 IU) can take the misery out of the menses. Take it in the morning, right after breakfast.

To Bring On Your Period: Dissolve one tablespoon of hot mustard powder in a cup of just-boiled water and add it to your bath water. Sit in the bath for twenty minutes, then rinse off under the shower. A mustard bath has been known to bring on a period.

To Slow the Flow: Raspberry leaf tea—a cup after each meal and one at bedtime—can help decrease your menstrual flow.

Prepare it as you would the yarrow tea (see above). It can also ease crampiness and the pain of swollen breasts. Raspberry tea is available at health food stores.

For All Menstrual Problems: Suma is an herb that comes in capsule form, is available at health food and vitamin stores, and is said to be an adaptogen—correcting whatever needs to be corrected. Follow the dosage on the label.

Gem Therapy: Chrysocolla, an exquisite rich blue/green opaque stone, definitely has female energy, according to gemologist Connie Barrett. In fact, it's recommended for men who want to get in touch with their feminine side.

Wear chrysocolla around your neck, carry it with you, or tape it on the problem area as you meditate, do a visualization, or say an affirmation.

♪ **Affirmation:** Repeat this affirmation ten times, first thing in the morning, each time you comb or brush your hair, and last thing at night—

I accept myself as a healthy and happy woman, blessed with normal and natural bodily functions.

More females than males suffer from motion sickness, and mostly between the ages of two and twelve. But plenty of adults are troubled with it. In fact, seventy-five percent of all astronauts experience some form of motion sickness.

Meanwhile, back on Earth . . . here are some suggestions for preventing or curbing this unpleasant condition:

• Twenty minutes before you board a plane or any other form of transportation, mix a half teaspoon of ginger powder in a glass of water and drink it. Or, take two capsules of powdered ginger.

Think of the leading over-the-counter motion sickness drug. This ginger remedy has been tested and found more effective than that drug . . . and without any of the side effects.

• This falls under the remedy category, you-may-think-this-is-crazy-but-it-seems-to-work. Before you start on your journey, tape a copper penny in your navel.

• Place a can of ice-cold beer behind your left ear, resting on your neck. Come to think of it, an ice-cold can of soda, juice—*anything*—will help prevent motion sickness.

• Help stave off motion sickness by putting on *airs*. On a plane, open the overhead vent; in a car, train, or bus, be sure to open a window; on a boat, stay on deck.

• Take the middle three fingers of one hand and put them on the inside of your wrist of the other hand, starting at the crease that separates the hand from the wrist. The center of your wrist, right after the fingers, is the pressure point that can prevent motion sickness. If you press that point while that hand is relaxed, your fingers should curl in. If that happens, you know you have the correct pressure point.

In order for this remedy to work, you have to exert constant pressure on that point. One way to do that is to put a button on the pressure point and a sweatband on your wrist to hold the button in place. For a similar commercial product on the market, check health food stores, boating shops, or the Magellan Catalogue (see RESOURCES for their listing).

Ground Motion Sickness Prevention: Before starting out, drape a black and white newspaper over your shoulders as though it were a beauty parlor cape. The smell of the paper and ink should help whether you're in a car, bus, or train.

How to Spell Relief Anywhere: When you're feeling queasy, on a plane or on the ground, relief is just a kitchen, bar, or newsstand away.

• Suck on a wedge of lemon. Once you're feeling better, rinse your mouth; the lemon is not good for teeth enamel.

• Drink a glass of papaya or pineapple juice.

• Eat a bowl of vegetable soup with a quarter of a teaspoon of cayenne pepper in it—half a teaspoon if you can stand it that hot.

• Eat two or three olives.

• Smell a black and white newspaper. Yes, take deep whiffs and catch up on current events at the same time.

The Best Place to Sit: In a plane, sit toward the front, or over the wheels. Do not sit in back of the plane. The tail moves more than the middle or front.

In any form of transportation, always sit near a window and look out; focus on things far away, not the nearby sights that are whizzing by.

The Best Time to Travel: Travel after dark and lower the odds of getting sick. When you fly by night, you can't see the unsettling motion as much as you do during daylight travel.

MUSCLE PAINS, SPRAINS, STRAINS, AND CRAMPS

Do you carry an attaché case in the same hand every day? On which side do you carry groceries? A pocketbook? A baby? Once you become aware of your daily toting pattern, you may realize why you have muscle pain in certain parts of your body. The remedy is obvious: Retrain yourself to keep shifting packages (or little people) from one side to the other.

Endorphins are the body's natural painkiller. Capsaicin, a substance found in red-hot peppers, is said to stimulate and increase the production of endorphins. Conclusion: Incorporate red-hot peppers into your diet to help you handle the pain.

SPRAINS AND STRAINS

• For most sprains and strains, especially if accompanied by pain and swelling, the word to remember is *RICE.* With us, this could mean that you prepare brown rice and . . . but no! In this case each letter stands for part of the treatment: *R* for rest—keep the injured body part still, *I* for ice—use an ice bag or a plastic bag with a towel around it, ten minutes on/ten minutes off throughout the day, *C* for compression—bind the sore muscle with an Ace bandage, and *E* for elevation—keep it raised.

• Take an egg white and mix in enough salt to form a thick paste. Gently massage the sore area with the paste. Don't wash it off until you're ready to repeat the procedure in two hours.

• Heat up three ounces of water and dissolve a tablespoon of salt in it. Then add three ounces of white vinegar. Dip a white washcloth into the solution, wring it out, and wrap it around the sore area. When the cloth starts drying, re-dip it and re-wrap it.

- To relieve the pain of a sprain and reduce the swelling, warm a cup of apple cider vinegar, then soak a piece of bread in it, and place the bread on the sore area. Put a piece of plastic over it and a towel over that. Keep it that way for 4 hours.

- This is useful if pain and swelling accompany a sprained or strained muscle: Grate an onion, or put it through the food processor. (See HEALTHFUL AND HELPFUL HINTS to learn to handle onions tearlessly.) Take the gratings, put it on the sore or swollen area, and wrap it around with plastic wrap.

- Relax in a bay leaf bath to soothe strained muscles. Put a half-cup of bay leaves in a pint of just-boiled water. Cover and let it steep for twenty minutes. Strain—not you, the bay leaves—and pour the liquid into your nice warm bath. Sit in the tub for at least fifteen restful minutes.

LEG CRAMPS
AND OTHER MUSCLE SPASMS

Calcium can be the answer for your muscle problems. Eat foods that are rich in calcium—green leafy vegetables, sesame seeds, and almonds. Drink fresh carrot juice. It contains calcium lactate that can do you a world of good.

Also, it may be a good idea to take calcium tablets. Since magnesium helps the absorption of calcium, you should consider tablets combining the two minerals. Depending on your size and the severity of your condition, take 800 to 1,500 mgs of calcium daily. It is important to consult your doctor to determine the appropriate dosage for you. While the pain is intense, your doctor may recommend low-dosage tablets at two-hour intervals, adding up to whatever daily dosage (s)he prescribes.

Relieve Leg Cramps: Take a piece of silverware—a spoon is best and it doesn't have to be silver, stainless steel is fine—and keep it by your bedside. When you awaken with a leg cramp, put the spoon on the cramp and it will uncramp instantly.

Wear socks to bed all year 'round and, we were assured by the person who shared this remedy with us, you'll never have another leg cramp. The socks can be heavy or light—they're all effective.

Swimmer's Leg Cramps: When you get a cramp and you're in the water, pinch your philtrum. Don't tell me you don't know what a philtrum is. It's the space between the upper lip and the nose. Grab hold of that little fleshy area from side to side and pinch! The leg will uncramp.

Toe Cramps: When your toes cramp, simply force yourself to point the toes toward your knee. Do it and the toes will uncramp.

Gem Therapy: Malachite is an exotic green stone with a pattern of swirls on it and is thought to be able to draw out pain. We were told that this somewhat expensive stone should be the size of the painful spot. If you have muscle pain throughout your body, you don't want to have to buy a malachite boulder, so forget this remedy. If your pain is very localized, place the stone on the exact spot and stay that way for fifteen minutes. That may be a good time to say the affirmation.

♪ **Affirmation:** Repeat this affirmation fifteen times a day, starting first thing in the morning and whenever a song pops into your mind, or when you hear music—

Energy flows through my muscles, making it easy to move to the music I love.

Neuropathy is the general term for a disorder of one or more nerves of the body. An inflammation of a nerve is *neuritis.* When the condition is accompanied by pain, it's called *neuralgia.* The most common type of neuropathy is an inflammation of the fifth cranial nerve that causes severe pain on one side of the face. It's called trigeminal neuralgia or *tic douloureux.* That's it for Anatomy 101.

Neuralgia can be caused by dental problems. If you've been diagnosed by a doctor and checked out by a dentist and still have neuralgic pain, you may want to try these suggestions—

• Massage fresh lemon juice on the painful areas and immediately follow up by placing hot, wet, white washcloths on the same areas.

• A poultice of hops (available at health food stores) can help bring quick relief from pain. Put a half cup of hops in cheesecloth. Leaving room for the hops to expand, tie the cheesecloth securely so that none of the hops can hop out. Dip the poultice in just-boiled water for two minutes. Shake off the dripping water, and when it cools off enough to apply without burning the skin, do it! Put it on the neuralgic spots with a dry towel on top to keep the heat in. As soon as it's no longer warm, reheat the poultice by re-dipping it in hot water.

• To help eliminate facial pain, all you may *knead* is a nine-minute massage. Using a circular motion, gently massage camomile oil (available at most health food stores) on the nape of the neck, the temples, and the sinus areas for three minutes each. Notice how just one drop of oil will go a long way.

- Bake a potato, cut it in half, and when it's cool enough, place both halves face down on the painful areas. To keep the heat in, cover them with a towel. Baked potatoes have been known to draw out neuralgic pain. We've also heard that a mashed potato poultice can do the same thing. No, not one report of relief from french fries.

- Grate about three ounces of horseradish root and mix it with about one tablespoon of white vinegar. After it marinates for an hour, spread it on the painful side of your face, particularly on your temple. Relax that way for twenty minutes. You may want to say the affirmation below during that time.

Prevention: According to old German preventive folk medicine, if you eat a large portion of raw sauerkraut daily, you will not be troubled with neuralgia.

♪ **Affirmation:** Repeat this affirmation fifteen times throughout the day, starting first thing in the morning, whenever you touch anything that's warm, and last thing at night—
Love fills me with happiness, harmony, and healing energy.

NOSEBLEED

Attention: If blood is flowing from both nostrils, it may not be just a simple nosebleed. You should get professional medical help immediately.

For the average, one-nostril nosebleed, sit up, calm down, and find the remedy that works for you. Here are some suggestions—

• Pack and pinch! First, gently blow your nose to clear out all the blood you can, making it easier to clot. Then pack your nose with a cotton ball. You can use a dry cottonball, or you can dip it in white vinegar or distilled witch hazel. Once the cotton ball is in the nostril, pinch together the fleshy part of your nose— gently but firmly—and stay that way for six to eight minutes.

If your nose is still bleeding, do the whole process one more time.

• Take off the outer shell of a bulb of garlic, then crush the bulb to a paste. Sculpt the paste into a pancake the size of a silver dollar. If your *right* nostril is bleeding, put the garlic pancake on the instep of the bottom of your *left* foot. If your *left* nostril is bleeding, put the garlic pancake on the instep of the bottom of your *right* foot.

• Hands seem to play an important part in stopping a nose-bleed. Submerge your hands in hot water, or raise your hands over your head, or raise the arm on the same side as the nostril that's bleeding, hold it stiff, and put that hand against the wall. Then lean on it.

• While you soak your feet in a basin of hot water, drink cayenne tea—one-eighth teaspoon in a big mug of warm water.

• If you're outdoors, clean off a leaf and place it under your upper lip. If there are no leaves around, place a dime under your lip or a piece of brown paper bag.

Prevention: It is said that a daily cup of yarrow tea (available at health food stores) will keep you free of nosebleeds. Most herbs have more than one name. Yarrow is also known as "soldier's woundwort," "old man's pepper," "knight's milfoil," and "nosebleed."

❧ Pets . . . Keeping ❧ Them Healthy

FOR DOGS AND CATS

Tune in to your pet to evaluate his needs. Use common sense when determining treatment dosage, taking into account the size of your pet. After treatment, pay careful attention to your pet's reaction. As with humans, if symptoms persist, seek professional help.

Diarrhea: Mix one teaspoon of carob powder (available at health food stores) in a glass of water and give it to your pet in the morning and the evening. If your pet's condition is not abating, give him the carob powder in water several times a day.

Ear Mites: When your pet seems to have itchy ears, take a flashlight and look inside them. If you see crud in the ear that resembles coffee grounds, chances are your pet has mites. Puncture vitamin E capsules, squeeze out the oil into each of your pet's ears, and gently rub it in. Then take cotton swabs and carefully clean out the oil along with the coffee grounds. Repeat the process three days in a row. The vitamin E oil will suffocate the mites and help heal the itchy ears.

Fleas: Since fleas are such a big problem for pet owners, we asked New Age–thinking veterinarians, animal trainers, and animal groomers how they take care of their own pets. All agreed that they never use chemical flea collars or sprays on their pets. Some collars and sprays are said to contain very strong ingredients that can cause all kinds of physical problems including heart trouble, allergies, and nervous system disorders.

There are *herbal* flea collars available at some pet shops and some health food stores.

Do-It-Yourself Flea Collar: Find a durable and comfortable collar—a leather strap or heavy-but-smooth twine—and soak it in pennyroyal oil (available at health food stores) for twenty-four hours. Then tie it around your pet's neck and fleas will flee.

Caution: Do not use pennyroyal if you or your pet are pregnant. In rare instances, it has caused cats to abort.

Removing Flea Eggs: Make a quart of strong pennyroyal tea. Sponge down your pet with the solution once a week for a month. After the sponging, take pennyroyal oil, mix one teaspoon in two ounces of water (for a large dog; half the amount for smaller dogs and cats), and gently rub it on your pet's coat.

The tea sponging should destroy fleas' eggs and the oil should repel fleas. The scent of the pennyroyal may also repel your pets, but they get used to it.

Caution: Do not use pennyroyal if you or your pet are pregnant. In rare instances, it has caused cats to abort.

Flea Repellents: Yes, fleas have a keen sense of smell. Here are more remedies known to successfully assault their little noses.

Cut two lemons into small bite-sized pieces, and place in a quart of water—peel and all. After it boils for an hour, take it off the burner and let it steep overnight. In the morning, strain and use the liquid to sponge down or spray your pet. While *fleas* will be repelled by the smell of citrus oil, the people who live with the pet find it pleasant. The lemon water will also help heal flea bites on your pet's skin.

Your pet's diet is said to play the most effective role in repelling fleas, specifically the addition of vitamin B-1 (thiamine) to the menu. Brewer's yeast (available at health food stores), a rich source of B-1, is highly recommended. Daily dosage gauge: one rounded tablespoon for fifty pounds of pet.

The way it's thought to work is that vitamin B-1 produces an odor that comes out on your pet's skin. We can't smell it, but it supposedly sickens the fleas.

To prevent brewer's yeast from causing gas, feed it to your pet in moist food and in small amounts.

Pet owners: You might also want to take a daily dose of brewer's yeast to protect yourselves from fleas.

Garlic, wouldn't you know, is another repellent. We heard about someone who rubs vegetable oil on his dog's skin, then massages in some garlic powder. True, the poor pet smells like a salami sandwich for a few hours, but because of the garlic, he's flea-free for a few months.

Experts agree—raw garlic is great for pets, whether they have fleas, worms, coughs, constipation, indigestion, whatever. Finely mince one to three cloves of garlic (depending on your pet's size) and add it to his food. If your pet has a problem with it, try garlic powder or oil.

Fleas hate the smell of cedar. See that your pet's living quarters contain cedar shavings or chips. For Christmas, buy your pet a cedar chest.

If you have an outdoor doghouse, put fresh pine needles in the house.

Ridding Your Home of Fleas: Fleas breed and hatch in carpeting and on furniture. Every other day, vacuum the areas where your pet hangs out and sleeps. Put on a pair of white socks and slowly walk through your home. Fleas will be attracted to your body warmth and electromagnetic energy. When they jump on your feet, the white socks will make them easy to see. Then get out the vacuum cleaner!

To make sure you kill the fleas and eggs that you suck up in the vacuum cleaner, place some chemical flea powder (the strong kind that you would *not* use on your pet) in the bag *before* vacuuming.

You can also sprinkle brewer's yeast on the carpeting, furniture, and other pet hang-outs.

Once a week, wash your pet's bedding.

Itching: To give your pet relief from an itch, dab on some apple cider vinegar.

Nurturing with Crystals: According to Joyce and Connie, proprietors of Crystal Gardens in New York City, animals respond to stones just as humans do. They had a cat and wanted to bring home a kitten. To avoid going through the usual long and unpleasant "getting used to each other" period, Joyce put rose quartz—a stone of nurturing and love—all around, including where the cats slept. In only two days, the older cat was mothering the kitten.

Caution: Be sure each stone you use is big—too big for your pet to swallow.

Pet/Owner Bonding: By encouraging your pet to eat the last few crumbs on your plate, it is said that you are attuning him to your vibes and strengthening his relationship with you.

Daily Health-Giving Diet for Cats and Dogs: As you may have already noticed, the remedies in this book are simple and easy to do. That's because we know how people are when it comes to their own health. But when it comes to the well-being of their pets . . . That's why we've included this recipe that Andi Brown, expert in Animal Nutrition, graciously shared with us for all of you who care for cats and/or dogs. It's called SPOT'S STEW, named for Andi's black and white longhair cat. When Andi adopted him, he had horrendous health conditions (too numerous and unpleasant to mention). Four days after being on this stew, Spot started to show great improvement, and a few weeks later, still on the stew, made a wonderful recovery.

Ingredients for Spot's Stew

2 onions, chopped coarsely
³⁄₄ head of garlic (not just 1 clove, but a "head")
1 whole fryer chicken (smallish)
16 oz. brown rice
handful of broccoli, cut up
4 carrots
1 whole zucchini
1 whole yellow squash
handful of green beans
2 stalks of celery

In a 10-quart stock pot (stainless steel, *please*) put 2–3 table-spoons of vegetable oil. Heat oil and then brown the onion and garlic lightly. Add the chicken, bones, skin, and all. Fill pot with water to cover chicken. Add brown rice, vegetables, and more water to cover. Cook over a low to low-medium heat for about 3 hours. After the stew has finished cooking, let it cool and then debone the chicken. Then take an electric hand mixer and mix the chicken, rice, and vegetables into a purée.

Using ziplock bags or small, empty milk cartons, package up meal-sized portions, and freeze what you don't need immediately. Seek your pet's advice for ideal meal size! (Andi makes up enough food to last a month.)

FOR DOGS: Add 1 slice of whole grain bread to each meal.

Andi also adds a blend of cold pressed oils (Dream Coat) to provide the essential fatty acids which are missing once these ingredients have been cooked, and a blend of water-soluble vitamins (Anitra's Vita-Mineral Mix) also missing from the cooked dish.

Skunk Odor Removal: If your pet gets sprayed by a skunk, put on rubber gloves and bathe him in tomato juice. You'll need a lot of tomato juice even though you can dilute it with water.

Or: It might be more economical to bathe your pet in vinegar diluted with water—one part vinegar to ten parts water. *Being careful not to get the solution in his eyes,* sponge his face with the vinegar. Do not rinse off the vinegar with water. The smell will return. Even by letting the vinegar dry naturally on him, you may have to give your pet one more treatment before the smell is gone forever.

Traveling with a Pet: Starting a few days before you travel with your pet, put three or four drops of peppermint oil in his/her water. Remember to pack the peppermint oil, so that when you're traveling you can continue putting it in your pet's water. That way, it will smell familiar and away-from-home water won't upset your pet and make him/her unwilling to drink it.

Worms: It's unanimous—garlic gets rid of worms and eggs, and prevents them from returning. Use common sense when it comes to dosage. One clove of garlic a week seems to be about right for puppies. Grown dogs, depending on size, should have two or three cloves a week.

Mince the garlic and mix it in your pet's food—a little at a time. A couple of garlic pills daily also seem to be effective wormers.

FOR DOGS ONLY

Arthritis and Lameness: Give your dog bone meal tablets. Start slowly—one a day for a medium-sized dog, and gradually regulate the dosage in accordance with his reaction and needs.

And/Or: Alfalfa tablets—three a day—have been known to make a dog's limp disappear.

Bad Breath: Mix some sprigs of fresh parsley into your pet's moist food, then add that to your pet's dry food. Once he downs it, his breath should be kissing sweet.

Cough: If your dog has a cough, give him a couple of garlic capsules every three hours until the cough subsides. And for Pete's sake, tell him he must stop smoking!

Diarrhea in Puppies: If your puppy has diarrhea, feed her cottage cheese for a couple of days—nothing else, just cottage cheese. It's an effective cure for this puppy condition called coccidiosis.

Ear Care: Once a week, dip a cotton ball in mineral oil and carefully wipe the insides of your dog's ears. This process helps prevent infection.

Note: Some breeds, like poodles and terriers, have hair growing inside the ear. Get a groomer to teach you how to pluck the ear hair to prevent wax and dirt from accumulating.

Eye Inflammation: If your dog loves to ride in the car with his head out the window, from time to time his eyes may get a little inflamed. Take a soft, lint-free cloth, dampen it, and carefully clean his eyes. Then drop a drop of castor oil in each eye. Do it twice a day until your dog's eyes are normal.

Feet—Protection When It Snows: Walking your dog on snowy sidewalks, strewn with commercial snow-melting products, can be dangerous to your dog's health. The chemicals in those products burn his paws. The dog licks his paws to soothe them, licking the chemicals that can make him sick. Right after you have walked your dog, wash his paws with a mixture of one teaspoon of baking soda to one glass of water. The baking soda solution will relieve the burning from the chemicals.

Gas: Rub apple cider vinegar on a dog's stomach—where the hair is sparsest—and within a half hour, the dog should be more socially acceptable company.

Keep Off: To train your young dog to stay off the couch and chairs, put sheets of aluminum foil on the seats. When your dog jumps up on it, *surprise!* The crumbling noise and the glare will frighten your pet into keeping her feet on the ground.

I said, *Keep Off!*: With Nancy Birnes's concoction from her book *Cheaper & Better* (Harper & Row, 1987), you can train your puppy to stay off the furniture and rugs. Mix one-fourth cup oil of cloves with one tablespoon of paprika and one teaspoon of black pepper. Pour the mixture into one of those stamp-moistener tubes and dab it all over furniture legs and around the edges of rugs. The scent will discourage the puppy from going where he's not wanted. If he isn't trained by the time the scent wears off, mix up another batch of the solution and reapply.

Not-Yet-Housebroken: If your puppy is still leaving puddles on your rug or carpet, put wheat germ on the wet area. It will dry leaving no stain and no smell. All you'll have to do is vacuum it up.

Shiny Coat: The addition of a couple of tablespoons of baking soda to your dog's bath and rinse water will make his coat soft and shiny.

Dry Skin: We heard about a dog who had chronic dry skin for years. Nothing helped, until the owner started mixing a tablespoon of safflower oil into the dog's food every day. A week later, the dry skin condition had cleared up completely.

Stop Shedding: If there's no end to your dog's shedding, massaging the coat with olive oil once a week has been known to limit the shedding to the appropriate seasons.

Teeth and Gums: Do not limit your dog's diet to soft foods. Canned food, table scraps, and other soft food do not clean tartar from the teeth. A build up of tartar can cause gum infection and soreness. Make sure your dog's diet is supplemented with dry food, hard dog biscuits, large bones, or some of my sister Joan's bran muffins.

FOR CATS ONLY

Cat Box Deodorizer: According to Nancy Birnes, author of *Cheaper & Better* (Harper & Row, 1987), to go a long time between litterbox changes, clean out the solid waste every day and add the contents of a sixteen-ounce box of baking soda to your kitty litter (four teaspoons of dried mint is optional), and stir it up often to aerate it.

Cuts and Scratches: Clean the wound with tepid water. (You may have to cut the hair to get to it.) Then puncture a vitamin E capsule and squeeze the oil onto the cut or scratch. Healing should start to take place without your being afraid that the cat will harm itself if it licks off the vitamin E. If that happens, just apply some more.

Food: We were told on good authority that a cat will not survive on a diet of dry dog food. A cat doesn't need all that bulk, but does need more vitamins and protein than dry dog food provides.

And: Put out a meal at a time for your cat, not more. Moist cat food that's left out half a day can sour, get moldy, or grow harmful bacteria that can seriously sicken your cat.

Also: Save the liquid from canned tuna fish for when your cat doesn't seem to like the food you're serving her. The tuna gravy may turn out to be the cat's meow.

Fur Balls: Make sure you feed your cat roughage—dry cat food or fresh grass—along with a daily teaspoon of vegetable oil, to enable him to pass the fur balls with the stools. Roughage and the daily dose of oil can help prevent large fur balls from forming.

Keep Off: If you have dark woodwork and a cat who likes to use it as a scratching post, get out the chili sauce. Cats are repelled by the smell of it. Rub the chili sauce on the woodwork, then buff it off and watch your cat stay away.

I Said, *Keep Off!*: To keep your cat off the couch or your favorite armchair, cram mothballs between the pillows, in the seams—wherever possible. Not too many or you won't want to sit there either.

Urinary Problem Prevention in Male Cats: Adding one teaspoon of white vinegar a day to your cat's water may help prevent the formation of stones that can eventually cause all kinds of urinary problems. A diet of low-ash cat food is also said to help.

FOR EXOTIC PETS

Canary—Sick and Moulting: Along with its regular seed feed, give the sick bird sponge cake that has been dipped in sherry. No matter how little of the sponge cake the bird eats, keep feeding it to him daily. We were told that this remedy, weird as it seems, can bring a canary back to health and fine voice in no time.

Cow—Cold: Did you know that cows catch cold? Add a tablespoon of black pepper to a quart of warm milk and give it to the cow. If you give a cow with a cold "milk," would you give a chicken that has a cold "chicken soup"?

Goat—Fly Repellent: Feed your goat a quarter of a cup of apple cider vinegar daily. Not only will they like the taste of it, but they'll love the results. It will keep flies away from them and even from their droppings.

Hens—Lice: Are your pet hens plagued with lice? A couple of times a week, mix three tablespoons of sulfur into their feed and the lice will lose their lease in the henhouse.

Horse—Shiny Coat: Add crushed oats to hay as part of the horse's diet, and his coat will get a lustrous sheen.

Parakeet—Fatigue: On a daily basis, add three drops of liquid vitamin C to the bird's drinking water and feed her blenderized sunflower seeds. Hopefully, you'll notice a difference in her energy level within a month.

Pigs—Worms: Coal—like the kind you find in your Christmas stocking if you've been naughty—worms pigs. Let your pig pig-out on a few chunks every now and then.

PET OWNER FOOD-FOR-THOUGHT

Have you noticed a correlation between what's going on in your life and your pet's illnesses?

Psychologist Lloyd Glauberman suggests, "Next time your pet is sick, take a good, long look at your present situation. Your emotional problems may be manifesting themselves in your pet. In some instances, the pet will not recover until its owner straightens out his or her life."

For your sake and the sake of your pet, lighten up so that both of you can thrive.

POISON IVY

We live in New York City and poison ivy is one of the few things neither of us ever worries about. However, when speaking to groups across the country and while doing radio and television shows, we're constantly asked for poison ivy remedies.

It's no wonder. Urushiol is the heavy oil in poison ivy that causes an allergic reaction. Plants with urushiol grow in every state except Alaska and Hawaii. Before you venture into areas that are most likely to have poison ivy growing, learn to recognize the three-leafed menace. Go to the library and find a book that has pictures of poison ivy. Take note of the thin, pale stems with three leaves on each stem.

Foremost world gardening authority Elvin McDonald shared with us this poison ivy poem from foliate folklore—

"Leaflets three, let it be."

The White Paper Test: If you think it's poison ivy but you're not sure, try the white paper test. Take hold of the plant with a piece of white paper and crush the leaves. If it's poison ivy, the juice on the paper will turn black in five minutes.

Getting Rid of the Plant: *Never* get rid of a patch of poison ivy by burning it. The plant's oil gets in the air and can be inhaled. You don't want poison ivy oil in your lungs. It can be very harmful. Instead, while wearing gloves, uproot the plants and leave them on the ground to dry out in the sun.

Or, prepare a solution of three pounds of salt in a gallon of soapy water. Spray the poison ivy plants over and over. If the solution doesn't do the trick, then drown 'em.

Note: Tools that are used for digging up poison ivy plants should be thoroughly washed with the (above) solution. When you're finished destroying the poison ivy and cleaning your tools, carefully take off your gloves, turning them inside out, and dispose of them. You may need to toss your clothes away also, since the poison ivy oil may not wash out completely and can stay active for at least a year.

POISON IVY REMEDIES

• The natural antidote is jewelweed (ironically also known as Spotted Touch-Me-Not). Of course, as you must learn to recognize poison ivy, you must also know what jewelweed looks like. So while you're in the library . . .

Jewelweed almost always grows right near poison ivy. Mother Nature—what a gal! There are several ways to use the jewelweed plant:

—Ball up the whole plant and use it to wipe the poison ivy oil off the skin.

—Crush the leaves and stem, releasing the juices, and apply it to the rash every hour throughout the day.

—Prepare a solution to keep on hand. Pick the whole plant and break it into small pieces. Cover it with at least a quart of water and let it boil until the water is a dark orange. Strain the liquid into a jar, cover it, and refrigerate until needed.

• If you realize you just brushed up against poison ivy and you can get to cold water within three minutes, you can wash away the nasty oil. *Do not use soap.* One theory is that the oil from the soap can seal in the poison ivy oil and the other theory is that the soap will remove the acid mantle that protects the skin.

• Take watermelon—both the rind and the meat of the melon—and glide it over and over the rash-ridden body parts. Let it dry naturally. Within a day, the condition should improve greatly.

- Aloe vera to the rescue! Every home should have an aloe vera plant. To help heal a poison ivy rash, take a small piece of the plant, squeeze out the gel, and apply it to the affected areas.

- Puncture a vitamin E capsule, squeeze out the oil, and apply that to the rash.

- Until you pick up an aloe vera plant or a bottle of vitamin E, apply olive oil to the rash.

- Make a paste of cornstarch and water, baking soda and water, or oatmeal and water. Put it on the rash for temporary relief from the itching.

- Pre-prepare this remedy: Make a quart of strong mugwort tea. (Mugwort is available at health food stores.) Bottle it and keep it in the refrigerator. The second you realize you have poison ivy, get the mugwort tea and wash the skin. If done quickly enough, you can remove the rash-causing oil from the skin. *Never* use warm mugwort tea. It will open the pores, allowing the oil to sink in.

- Dip white washcloths into a pint of buttermilk, with or without a tablespoon of salt mixed in, and apply the cloths to the affected areas. Keep dunking and re-applying. Then, after the last dunk, let it dry naturally. The buttermilk should help bring down swelling, stop running sores, and dry up the rash.

Resistance-Builder: Eating romaine lettuce daily for two weeks before being exposed to poison ivy is said to help build one's resistance to it.

Prevention: A woman in the Midwest shared this with us, saying that it works for her and her family. Neither of us has tested this, so you're on your own. Proceed with caution.

Wet a washcloth with whiskey, rub your exposed body parts with it before going into poison ivy-infested areas, and contact with poison ivy will not affect you.

Immunization: First, get a goat. Did I lose you or are you still with me? Have the goat graze where there is poison ivy. It will not harm the goat. After the goat has eaten the poison ivy, put on gloves and, making sure all your body parts are covered, milk the goat. Throw that milk away. The *second* milking—ah, that's the important one. Drink at least a pint of milk from the second milking and it will immunize you for a year.

Rent-a-Goat. How's that as an idea for a business? *No kidding!*

POISON OAK

Poison oak is to the West Coast what poison ivy is to the eastern part of the country. The consensus of opinion is that the remedies for poison ivy are also effective for poison oak sufferers.

PREGNANCY...
AND RIGHT AFTER

Pregnancy is a very personal experience. What's true for one mother-to-be may not be so for another. For that reason, it's most important to check with your obstetrician before you adopt any of the suggestions in this chapter.

STARTING OUT THE HEALTHY WAY

Avoid the Risk of Miscarriage: Stop smoking! In women who smoke, it is estimated that miscarriages occur in about twenty-five out of a hundred pregnancies.

For those with a history of miscarriage, sage tea—two cups a day—seems to be the "sage" drink to have.

Prevent Allergies in Baby: Throughout your pregnancy, do not overload on any one food item. During at least the last three months of pregnancy, do not eat foods to which you're allergic, and you can avoid passing along that allergy to your baby. Even while nursing, stay away from those foods.

Minimize Stretch Marks: Get out the sesame oil. Rubbing the oil on your body every day can let the skin stretch at its own pace and help prevent subsequent stretch marks.

For a Tear-free Delivery: To enhance elasticity and lessen the chances of tearing during childbirth, oil the opening to the vagina every day during pregnancy, using sesame oil. This remedy gives new meaning to the phrase, "Open Sesame!"

For an Easier Pregnancy/Faster Delivery: Even some obstetricians are prescribing this—raspberry leaf tea. The herb has vitamins A, C, B, and E, also calcium, phosphorus, iron, and more good stuff that can help prevent miscarriages, curb morning sickness, reduce labor pains, and make for an easy, fast delivery.

Some herbalists think it best to drink a cup or two of raspberry leaf tea every day of your pregnancy. Others feel it's okay to start drinking the tea in the sixth month. Still others believe that women need only have the tea the last six weeks of the pregnancy.

Preparation also varies considerably. The recipe we like best is used in Chinese medicine: Pour one pint of just-boiled water over two rounded teaspoons of dried raspberry leaves (available at health food stores and in bulk at herb shops). Let it steep for a half hour. Strain and drink it throughout the day. In cold weather, you may want to warm it up a little before drinking.

Or try Squawvine. Doesn't the name of this trailing evergreen make you feel as though—once you drink the tea made from the herb—you go out on the prairie, squat, and have your baby? Herbalists agree that it can help make childbirth a quick and easy experience.

Preparation and dosage of Squawvine (available at herb shops) is the same as raspberry leaf tea (see above). In fact, you can combine the two herbs, a rounded teaspoon of each in a pint of just-boiled water, to make one extremely beneficial tea.

Stamina Booster for an Easier Birth: According to British childbirth writer Sheila Kitzinger, if you eat garlic and onions on a regular basis, starting in your third month, your stamina will increase, and birth will be easier. If you need a scientific reason to justify your anti-social breath, the linoleic acids in both garlic and onion help produce prostaglandins that help stimulate cervical effacement and dilation.

DEALING WITH MORNING SICKNESS

Morning sickness usually starts around the sixth week of pregnancy, peaks during the eighth and/or ninth weeks, and ebbs off after the thirteenth week.

Here's what you can do about it—

- Keep papaya juice (without any additives) or papaya concentrate in the refrigerator. A glassful of the juice or the diluted
concentrate can make you feel better quickly.

- Relief can be minutes away with yarrow tea. It works wonderfully well for some women. Add one heaping teaspoon to
one cup of just-boiled water. Let it steep for ten minutes. Strain
and drink.

- A lot of testing has been done with ginger powder for
motion sickness. The results have been impressive. Ginger
powder is more effective than the leading medicines on the
market—and with none of the side effects.

Ginger also seems to be effective for morning sickness. The
recommended dose is two capsules of powdered ginger root
before breakfast. Or simply make yourself a cup of tea by
steeping four quarter-size slices of fresh ginger root in a mug
of just-boiled water, for about ten minutes.

Caution: Use only with your doctor's approval!

- If you're having waves of nausea during the day when
you're out and about, eat raw almonds. One almond has more
protein content than beefsteak, is rich in calcium, potassium,
the B vitamins, vitamin E, plus other vitamins and minerals.
Don't leave home without them. Six to ten of 'em make a
healthy snack and can quell the queasiness. Bear in mind, however, that they are about forty-five percent fat.

AFTER BABY'S BIRTH

Getting in Shape: Asian tradition says that, after childbirth,
eating seaweed—kelp and dulse—one or two small portions a
day for a month, helps get the uterus back to its original size.

Promoting Your Milk Supply: Alfalfa tea, anise seed tea,
and dill seed tea (available at health food stores) are all said to
help ensure the supply of milk for the mom who is breast-
feeding.

To prepare the tea, steep a teaspoon of any of the above in
a cup of just-boiled water. After ten minutes, strain and drink
it before each feeding.

REFERRAL

For information about breast-feeding, write to or call:

La Leche League International, Inc.
1400 N. Meacham Road
P.O. Box 4079
Schaumburg, IL 60168-4079
800/525-3243

PROSTATE

The prostate is a chestnut-sized gland that men have. It's located alongside and under the bladder, surrounding the urethra.

There are two common prostatic problems: prostatitis—an inflammation of the prostate that can affect men thirty-something to middle-age; and, an enlarged prostate that may affect men over age sixty.

At the first sign of a prostate symptom—frequent urination, burning sensation while urinating, difficulty urinating—see your health professional. And since medical experts agree that coffee and alcoholic beverages are b-a-a-a-a-a-d for anyone with a hint of a prostate problem, eliminate those stimulants immediately.

To help prevent prostate trouble, see the suggestions below—

Prevention: The classic folk remedy for prostate health is eating a handful—at least an ounce—of raw, shelled pumpkin seeds daily. The seeds are rich in zinc. Don't be surprised to find that the pumpkin seeds give you more sexual vitality.

If you aren't going to eat the seeds every day, then supplement your diet with 25 to 50 mgs of zinc.

Caution: Prolonged use of zinc can cause a copper deficiency.

• There seems to be a strong statistical association between low vitamin A status and prostate cancer. Eat foods rich in vitamin A: broccoli, carrots, cauliflower, swiss chard, endive, kale, collard greens, mustard greens, dandelion greens, spinach, tomatoes, loose leaf lettuce, fish liver oil, winter squash, sweet potatoes, watercress, turnip greens, beet greens, cantaloupe, peaches, apricots, prunes, cherries, and papayas.

Vitamin A supplements can be toxic. They should be taken only under the supervision of a health professional.

• Pygeum Africanum extract comes in capsules of 50 mgs each and is available at most health food and vitamin shops. Take two or three a day to help prevent prostate trouble—or to help treat the onset of a prostate problem.

• It is said that cucumbers contain beneficial hormones. Nourish the prostate gland by eating a large cucumber daily.

• Drink a cup of oatstraw tea daily. Prepare the oatstraw (available at health food stores) by adding a teaspoon of the dried herb to a cup of just-boiled water. Let it steep for ten minutes. Strain and drink.

PROSTATE REMEDIES

• Bee pollen has been known to successfully treat prostate conditions. Once your doctor says it's okay to try this, start real slow with a few granules a day. If you have no allergic reaction to the bee pollen, gradually work your way up to taking two teaspoons a day. If you prefer taking tablets, then work your way up to four tablets a day. The granules and tablets are available at health food stores, or see RESOURCES for a reputable distributor.

Bee pollen, by the way, like pumpkin seeds, can also improve your sexual vitality.

• Saw palmetto berry tea has a sweet aromatic taste. Prepare it by steeping a heaping teaspoon of the herb in a cup of just-boiled water for seven minutes. Strain and drink three cups a day.

♪ **Affirmation:** Repeat this affirmation nine times a day—starting first thing in the morning, every time you look at your watch, and last thing at night—

I richly deserve all the good things in life—happiness, love, and the best of health.

Ringworm is not always ring-shaped and it isn't caused by worms. It's a common fungus infection that's very contagious. That's one reason you don't want to use anyone else's comb, brush, or towel. You can also get ringworm by petting infected dogs and cats. Once you have ringworm, you have to take care not to scratch the sore, scaly area. You can easily spread the parasite to other parts of your body.

Here are some remedies that can help clear up the condition—

• Put a copper penny in vinegar and keep it there until it turns green—the penny, not you. Then take the wet penny and rub it on the ringworm. The combination of the vinegar and greened copper is said to make it better. Repeat the procedure at least three times a day.

• Finely mince two cloves of garlic and mix them together with the oil from three punctured vitamin E (400 IU) capsules. Spread the mixture on the infected area three times a day to stop the itching and start the healing.

• Take a piece of paper from a child's notebook, roll it into a tube, and tie it in three places—top, middle and bottom. Carefully burn the tied tube in an ashtray. Apply the residue (technical term: brownish guck) on the ringworm every morning and evening until the sore patches are gone.

• This is one of those strange old remedies that sounds awful, seems awful, is awful, and works.

Take fountain pen ink—oh, about a thimble full—and mix it with cigar ashes—about ten flicks should do. Paint the mixture on the ringworm area and within three to four days the ring-worm has been known to completely clear up.

𝒮 **Affirmation:** Repeat this affirmation at least ten times, first thing in the morning, last thing at night, and each time you blame yourself or others for something—

I forgive myself and I forgive others. There's great harmony in my life now.

Sciatica is a swelling of or injury to the sciatic nerve, causing pain, soreness, or tingling. Since the sciatic nerve starts at the base of the spine and travels down the thigh and leg to the foot, the pain can be as extensive as the nerve.

In some cases, sciatic pain may be caused by a misalignment in the body. Professional help would then be needed to properly align your body.

Bed rest and heat—hot baths and heating pads—are usually recommended for sciatica, along with warmed castor oil or olive oil packs and massages.

We have additional suggestions for you to try after you check them with your health professional—

• A poultice of hops can bring fast relief for sciatic pain sufferers. Yes, the same hops used for making beer. In fact, the Spanish name for hops is, "flores de cerveza," which means "flowers of beer." Be warned, it doesn't smell like flowers and it doesn't smell like beer. Actually, the smell is rather unpleasant. But if it relieves the pain . . .

The poultice you're going to make, is to be placed directly on the sore area, so you're going to have to use your judgment as to how much of the herb to use, depending on the size of your painful area. You might start by steeping three tablespoons of hops in a cup of just-boiled water. After ten minutes, strain off the liquid, but don't throw it out, and put the moist hot hops in cheesecloth, wrapping it around to form a poultice. Put it on the painful area and keep it there until it cools off. Then heat up the hops water and pour it over the poultice, re-moistening and re-heating it. Once again apply the poultice while it's nice and hot—as hot as you can take it without burning your skin.

- Another effective massage mixture is ginger and sesame oil. Grate a chunk of fresh ginger root, or put it through a food processor. Then put the pulp in a piece of cheesecloth and squeeze out the juice into a container. Mix an equal amount of sesame oil with the ginger juice, then massage the mixture on the painful areas. There may be a burning sensation from the ginger. If you feel it's too strong, simply add more sesame oil.

- Vitamin E—one 400 IU daily—has been quite effective for many people with sciatica. You should notice results within a couple of weeks.

  Please note: Vitamin E is one vitamin where more is *not* better. Play it safe and check with your doctor before starting this treatment.

- Drink a cup of celery tea before each meal and at bedtime. Not only has it been known to relieve pain but, for some people, it actually clears up the condition. Dried celery is available at health food stores. Use a heaping teaspoon in a cup of just-boiled water and let it steep for ten minutes. Strain and drink.

Acupressure: Vigorously massage the little tuft at the base of your pinky, on the same side as the sciatic pain. Keep at it for at least six minutes. It can ease the pain considerably.

Aromatherapy: Jasmine, considered the symbol of sensuality, is also known to soothe sciatic pain. Mix a half-teaspoon of jasmine oil with two teaspoons of liquid lecithin (both available at health food stores) and massage the painful area.

Incidentally, the lecithin increases absorption into the skin.

♪ **Affirmation:** Repeat this affirmation at least fifteen times, before and after each meal and during any kind of treatment—drinking celery tea, massaging the base of the pinky, using a hops poultice, whatever—

I walk through life with joy and ease, safely doing whatever I please.

❧ SEXUAL PROBLEMS ❧

The most sexually active people in the world are supposedly the Mangaians of Polynesia. (Now *there's* a place to open a motel.) It has been reported that the average eighteen-year-old couple makes love three times a night, every night. About ten years later, at age twenty-eight, their sex life dwindles down to two times a night, every night. The report stopped there. The reporter was either too busy to do a follow-up, or just too tired.

In any case, we don't have to worry about the Mangaians. And we may not have to worry about you, once you check out some of these suggestions—

The Best Time for Sex—Day vs. Night: Research says that sunlight enhances one's sex drive. It has to do with the arousal of the pituitary gland, which regulates the ovaries and testes. And that happens during the brightest part of the day. The *lack* of daylight is a signal for the brain's pineal gland to produce melatonin, a substance that inhibits ovulation, sperm production, and hormones that are responsible for sexual desire.

Melatonin levels are five times higher at night. This may explain the popularity of the song "Help Me Make It Through the Night."

The Best Months for Sex: Studies show a direct correlation between men's highest levels of testosterone—the hormone that regulates their sex drive—and the months of optimum sunlight, which are in summer and early fall. When you're planning your vacation, keep in mind the fact that July is the month with the longest and sunniest days of the year. But don't travel to South America in July. It's winter there then and testosterone levels in men are lowest in the winter months.

Aromatherapy for Sexual Arousal: Fill the air with the essence of rose, vanilla, jasmine, ginger, tonka, pine, or ylang-ylang and it will fill your heart with lust. For industrial strength stimulation, dab a drop of any one of the oils right under your nose.

Stay away from lavender. It will make you feel like going to bed . . . for a good night's sleep.

Gem Therapy for Sexual Energy: The stone with the most sexual energy is the ruby. You don't have to have an expensive faceted gem. There are rough rubies that are fairly affordable and there are raw ruby crystals that are reasonably priced.

If rubies don't turn you on, you might turn to the carnelian. It's a very inexpensive orange stone, also known for its sexual energy.

For Sexual Stamina and Vitality: To extol the benefits of bee pollen, the title of Noel Johnson's book says it all: *A Dud at 70 . . . a Stud at 80!* (Plains Corporation, 1982).

Start with a few grains of bee pollen each day. After three days, if you don't have an allergic reaction to it, increase the dosage to a quarter of a teaspoon. Then, gradually work your way up to one or two teaspoons a day, depending on how you feel. Let your body be your guide.

Or try halvah, a sweet treat from the Middle East, which dates back to when Cleopatra was dating. It's said to be especially effective for women.

You can buy halvah, but the commercial product does not have the potency of halvah made by loving hands at home.

It's easy to prepare. Grind a cup of sesame seeds. Mix in raw honey until it's the consistency of firm dough. Then break off chunks and roll them into bite-size pieces and enjoy.

Sesame seeds and raw honey are a powerful combination of magnesium, calcium, potassium, lecithin, phosphorus, bee pollen, aspartic acid, and more. Partake of the confection and you'll want to partake of the affection.

ABOUT APHRODISIACS

The most effective aphrodisiac is your own passion. The second most effective aphrodisiac is said to be ground rhinoceros horn . . . or is it a horny rhinoceros on the ground?—whatever. There's talk that these are the third best aphrodisiacs—

• Damiana leaf extract (botanical name: turnera aphrodisiaca)—five to eight drops daily (available at most health food stores)

• Seaweed—daily portions of dulse or kelp

• Legumes—word has it that St. Jerome did not allow nuns to eat beans for fear they would cause the nuns to get into bad habits

• Hot spices

• Onions, scallions, garlic

• Asparagus, arugula, artichokes

• Banana, fresh figs, cherries, peaches

• Sunflower seeds—raw, shelled

• Foods rich in B vitamins: green leafy vegetables, fish, wheat germ, almonds, peanut butter—the kind you get in health food stores without additives or preservatives

IMPOTENCE IN MALES

It's important to determine whether the impotence you're experiencing is physical (perhaps a side effect of medication you're taking, or arteriosclerosis, or a high-fat diet), or psychological (maybe it's bedroom boredom, or the fear of failure). An estimated ninety percent of all cases are psychological and temporary.

The Stamp Test: Go to your local post office and buy a *roll* of postage stamps. When you go to sleep, put a band of stamps around the shaft of the penis. Tear off the excess stamps and tape the first and last stamp to each other—not loosely, but not too tight.

If your condition is psychological, you will have an average of five erections in your sleep. During an erection, when the penis enlarges, the perforations of one of the stamps should tear apart. If your impotency is physical, nothing will happen to the stamps overnight.

Put postage on your penis every night for a couple of weeks and, at the end of that time, you will know if your impotency is physical or psychological, by the regularity with which the stamps' perforations were split apart. If it's psychological, sometimes just knowing the *mechanism* is in good working order will relieve the anxiety and enable you to perform while you're awake.

If your impotence stems from a physical problem, work with a health professional to pinpoint the cause. You might want to try the following suggestions . . . with your doctor's supervision:

• Ginseng—an herb that will not fail ya', for conditions genitalia.

The *haiku* (Japanese lyric poem with seventeen syllables) reflects the confidence many herbalists have in the herb. Ginseng comes in many forms—tablets, capsules, powder, extract, and the fresh whole root. Some herbalists think that eating a small slice of the whole root every day is the most beneficial way to take ginseng. Then again, some herbalists opt for the herb in powder form. Go to a health food store or herb shop and see what's available. Read labels. Ask knowledgeable store personnel for their input. When you know what you want, check out your selection and the dosage with your health professional to make sure it's appropriate for you.

It probably took a while for your problem to manifest itself; it may take a while for you to get results. Be consistent and patient.

• True unicorn extract (available at most health food stores) has been known to help reverse impotency. Take five to eight drops in water every day.

- Prepare oatstraw tea (available at health food stores) by steeping two teaspoons of the herb in one cup of just-boiled water. After five minutes, strain; drink a cup for breakfast and a cup after dinner, daily.

- Take cold baths or cold showers as often as once a day, not less than four times a week. Be patient (that's easy for us to say)—it may take a couple of months for results.

- Add a handful of raw pumpkin seeds to your daily diet. While you're at it, also eat raw or roasted sesame seeds—two tablespoons a day. Wash it down with sarsaparilla tea (available at health food stores). The seeds and the tea are said to be sexual stimulants and help prevent prostate problems.

Impotence Prevention: Some Japanese practitioners advise their patients to squeeze their testicles on a daily basis, once for each year of their life. J. Walter Allen, a friend in Florida who just celebrated his ninety-seventh birthday, read about this preventive treatment and said, "There goes my day."

♪ **Affirmation to Help Overcome Impotence:** Repeat this affirmation seven times, starting first thing in the morning, every time you turn something on—a light switch, the TV, the VCR, the car ignition—and again, last thing at night.

I accept my sexuality as part of my healthy, functioning mind and body. I allow myself to experience complete fulfillment, getting and giving pleasure and joy.

FRIGIDITY IN FEMALES

Here are two frigidity remedies—

- What ginseng does for men, dong quai is said to do for women. This Chinese root comes in several forms including tablets, capsules, and extracts—all with recommended daily dosage on the labels. Check out your selection and the dosage with your health professional to make sure it's appropriate for you.

Please don't expect "instant thaw." It may take a while for results.

• A daily dose of potato juice can get the ol' juices going. Take a medium-sized potato, scrub it clean, and grate it or feed it into a food processor. Place the pulp on cheesecloth, squeeze out the juice, then bottoms up . . . uh, that is, drink the potato juice, then bottoms up!

♪ **Affirmation to Help Overcome Frigidity:** Repeat this affirmation seven times, starting first thing in the morning, every time you turn something on—a light switch, the TV, the microwave, the car ignition—and again, last thing at night.

I accept my sexuality as part of my healthy, functioning mind and body. I allow myself to experience getting and giving physical pleasure and joy.

INFERTILITY

During the average woman's reproductive years, she has about 450 eggs that can be fertilized. During one average man's ejaculation, his testes manufacture about 400 million sperm cells. If all of this is *inconceivable,* these suggestions may help—

FOR MEN AND WOMEN:

• Stop smoking! Studies show that cigarette smoking can affect men's fertility by lowering the sperm count and causing the sperm to have less mobility; women smokers may be less fertile because of altered hormone levels; also, spontaneous miscarriages occur much more often in smokers than in non-smokers.

• Relax! Stress in men can promote muscle spasms in the sperm ducts that would interfere with the transmission of semen. Stress in women can cause an enlarged uterus, can prevent ovulation, and can cause abnormal cervical secretions that immobilize sperm.

• Eat a portion of seaweed every day—dulse, kelp, wakame, nori, or any of the others. It is especially nourishing for the reproductive systems of both men and women.

• Eliminate green peas and yams from your diet. They contain estrogenic chemicals that are known to be anti-fertility agents.

FOR MEN ONLY:
• Take royal jelly—up to 1,000 mgs a day—to increase your sperm count and make them more aggressive.

• Eat raw carrots. They're rich in zinc, which is known to increase the sperm count. Non-domesticated rabbits eat few, if any, carrots and they don't reproduce nearly as frequently as the domesticated rabbits.

• Get rid of tight underwear. The production of sperm is best at below body temperature. Briefs hold the testicles closer to the body, raising the temperature in there. Okay, so boxer shorts aren't sexy, but they'll help keep you cool where it counts.

FOR WOMEN ONLY:
• If you need to use a lubricant for intercourse, then during the few days of the month when you're fertile, use an egg white. Commercial lubricants may interfere with the sperm's survival and mobility. Since the white of an egg is protein, and the sperm is mostly protein, the egg white will not hinder the sperm's potential. Use room-temperature egg white. It can be applied to the penis or the vagina.

• Overly acidic cervical secretions can kill the sperm. You can neutralize the acidic secretions by douching with baking soda and water right before intercourse.

• Take dolomite (available at health food stores) daily. This combination of calcium and magnesium can promote pregnancy. Follow the dosage on the label.

For whatever reason you turned to this chapter, and no matter what problem you may be experiencing, just remember the immortal words of Rodney Dangerfield who said, "If it weren't for pickpockets, I'd have no sex life at all!"

REFERRALS

For free information, a confidential consultation, and treatment referral for sexually transmitted diseases, all paid for by the federal government, call:

STD Hotline
8 AM–11 PM E.S.T. Mon–Fri
800/227-8922

For information on specific topics, access to databases, and a non-circulating library at a reasonable fee, and free referrals to organizations, write to or call:

SIECUS (Sexuality Information and Education Council of the U.S.)
130 West 42nd Street—Suite 350
New York, NY 10036
212/819-9770

SHINGLES
(HERPES ZOSTER)

The same virus that produces chicken pox in children causes shingles in adults.

The infected and inflamed nerve centers are usually accompanied by patches of blisters and intense pain, mostly affecting the chest, abdomen, and/or face.

The following suggestions can bring instant relief from pain and itching, and can even clear up the condition completely:

• The more we research the benefits of apitherapy—treatment using honeybee products—the more impressed we are with results.

To rid you of the pain of shingles and to help heal the lesions, smear bee propolis in liquid form on the sore area a few times throughout the day. Use a soft pastry brush or a rouge brush. Liquid propolis is available at some health food stores and through bee products distributors listed in RESOURCES.

Another bee product that's extremely healing is raw honey. Spend a few pennies extra if you have to, to get the *raw* stuff. Just like with the liquid bee propolis, spread the honey on the sore areas a few times throughout the day, and expect pain to disappear and lesions to start healing.

• If you have shingles on your chest, gently bind the affected area with an Ace bandage, particularly before going to bed. The small amount of pressure from the bandage can relieve the pain without hindering your breathing.

• If you have a juicer or a food processor, prepare fresh leek juice and apply it directly to the blistered areas for immediate relief of the itching.

• Prepare elderflower tea, available at most health food stores, by adding a teaspoon of the dried herb to a cup of just-boiled water. Cover the cup and let it steep for 4 to 6 minutes, then strain and drink. Herbalist Ann Warren-Davis says, "Drink it three or four times a day. I've known it to clear up shingles in a day or two."

• Throughout the day, puncture vitamin E capsules and squeeze out the oil on the blisters. It stops the itching and, in some case, brings about a complete cure.

• Shingles is one of many problems that can be helped by the gel of the aloe vera plant. When using the plant, start with the bottom leaves first; they're the oldest. Either peel away the top layer of the leaf's skin and spread the gel on your skin, or cut off a piece of leaf and squeeze out the gel. For many, aloe means instant relief.

♪ **Affirmation:** Repeat this affirmation twelve times, starting first thing in the morning, right after applying anything to the sore lesions, and last thing at night—

I am relaxed and surrounded by positive energy as my body heals itself.

Sinus conditions can be caused by weather changes, by air conditioning, by an overheated room, by allergies, by gosh—anything, including dust that collects in one's mustache. It's up to you to discover your sinus triggers. It's up to us to give you suggestions that may help alleviate sinus symptoms. Here are some for congestion—

• During a sinus attack, chew a one-inch square of honeycomb (available at most health food stores). After you swallow the honey, continue chewing the waxy gum for about ten minutes. It can help stop the sneezing, clear up the congestion, and give you a spurt of energy, too.

• An old folk remedy for dissolving mucus is fenugreek seed tea (available at health food stores). When your sinuses need to be drained, prepare the tea by steeping a teaspoon of the fenugreek seed in a cup of just-boiled water. After seven minutes, strain and drink.

• In the Orient, the leaves of the ginkgo bilboa tree have been used as medicine for over 2,800 years. Now that the hearty ginkgo trees are popular in America, we are discovering the medicinal value of their beautiful fanlike leaves. They can help relieve sinus congestion. Crush a handful of the leaves, boil them, and carefully inhale the vapor. If you don't have the fresh leaves, ginkgo can be bought in capsule form. Follow the recommended dosage on the label.

• According to Dr. Nicholas Murray from the University of Melbourne in Australia, an ice pack applied to the bridge of the nose and across the cheek bones shrinks inflamed tissues.

• At the onset of sinus symptoms, Dr. Andrew Weil advises using hot wet towels on your upper face. The hotter the better, without burning yourself, of course. Keep the towels hot, wet, and on your face for fifteen minutes at a time, three or four times a day. It will promote drainage and increase blood flow to the area.

• Inhaling salt water is the classic folk remedy for sinus problems. It's been around for hundreds of years simply because it works.

Dissolve one-quarter teaspoon of salt (some people prefer to use sea salt) in one cup of warm spring or distilled water. (Tap water may have contaminants, including chlorine, that can further aggravate your sinus condition.)

The object of this is to inhale the salt water solution through your nostrils—one side at a time—have it go down toward your throat, and spit it out of your mouth rather than swallow it. This is not a pleasant procedure at first, but you will get used to doing it and it sure is effective.

You can pour the salt water into your cupped hand, close one nostril, and inhale through the open nostril, or you can use a medicine dropper or a small cup with a spout designed especially for this purpose and available at health food stores. In any case, you have to tip your head back and then spit the solution out of your mouth. After you've inhaled through both nostrils a few times, gently blow your nose.

You may cough the first few times you do it, but force yourself to continue. It gets a lot easier and you may even get to the point where you look forward to doing it. For congestion and inflamed tissues, do it once or twice a day.

If you have a sinus infection, use this salt water treatment two to four times a day to speed up the healing.

Reflexology for Sinus Congestion and Headache: Use the inside top half of your thumb, or a teaspoon to apply pressure on the roof of your mouth. This reflexology remedy can help make your headache disappear as it breaks up congestion.

Acupressure for All Sinus Symptoms: Vigorously massage the base of your three smallest toes. Within minutes, you should feel the sinus passages open. Once that happens, end the treatment by massaging the base of the big toes for two or three minutes.

♪ **Affirmation:** Repeat this affirmation twelve times, starting first thing in the morning, every time you pick up a tissue, and last thing at night—

I breathe easy knowing I am surrounded by positive energy, healing feelings, and people who love me.

Skin is one of our body's largest and heaviest organs. The average adult's skin measures nineteen square feet and weighs about nine pounds. The thinnest sections of skin are on your eyelids; the thickest are on your palms and the soles of your feet.

The average person sheds about a pound-and-a-half of skin particles each year. By the time you're seventy, you will have lost a little over a hundred pounds of outer skin. Those shedded skin particles are replaced with another coat of skin about once a month. And you say you have nothing new to wear!

There are close to 1,000 diseases and conditions that can affect our skin. In this chapter, we're going to deal with the dozen or so most common skin problems, starting with—

Acne: Using a jar with a cover, prepare this acne solution. Put eight ounces of water in the jar, then add ten drops of bee propolis extract (available at most health food stores or check RESOURCES). Dip a cotton ball into the solution, then dab the acne area with it. Start first thing in the morning and continue throughout the day whenever you can. Be sure to apply the solution after each time you wash your face and at bedtime. Be consistent and do it every day for at least three weeks, unless the acne clears up before that.

• Or, use aloe vera juice (available at health food stores) to help heal acne. With a cotton ball, dab it on first thing in the morning and last thing at night. If possible, apply it throughout the day, especially after you wash your face. Be consistent and do it every day for at least three weeks, unless the acne clears up before that.

- This has been reported to us as a "when all else failed, as a last resort" remedy. Take your first urine of the day on a white washcloth and pat it on the acne area. Or, if there's an infant around, use the baby's wet diaper. Urine is said to have our body's antibodies that are very healing. Be consistent. Do it daily. If you're not too grossed out, do it more than once a day.

- Drink three to four cups of stinging nettle tea a day. Prepare the tea with a teaspoon of the herb in a cup of just-boiled water. Let it steep for ten minutes. Strain and drink. Stinging nettle is known to help heal several skin problems including acne.

- For complexion perfection, think zinc! Eat foods rich in zinc—whole grains, sunflower seeds, pumpkin seeds (get them shelled and raw at health food stores), beans, spinach, mushrooms, brewer's yeast, and wheat germ. Of course you can supplement your diet with zinc tablets, but do so with the guidance of a health professional. Prolonged use of zinc can cause copper deficiency.

- For acne scars, put pieces of fresh pineapple on the acne scars and leave them there for fifteen minutes a day.

  Or, puncture a vitamin E capsule and squeeze out the oil on the acne scars. Do this at least an hour before going to bed, after you've washed your face for the night. Be consistent and patient. It may take quite a while before you see results.

  If you want to try both remedies, use the pineapple right after dinner and the E oil close to bedtime.

Age Spots: These brown patches we call *age spots* are caused by changes in pigmentation in sun-exposed areas of skin. They are also (wrongly) referred to as liver spots. The liver has nothing to do with the formation of the spots.

To be spotless, rub the patches with a slice of red onion for two or three minutes at a time, at least twice a day. Be consistent and patient for results.

Incidentally, the correct medical term for these patches is *lentigines.*

- The treatment that promises to be the fastest age spot remover is one using fresh pineapple juice. The key word is *fresh* . . . not canned, jarred, bottled, frozen, powdered, or concentrated. If you want the bromelain enzyme to get in there and help dissolve those spots, we're talking FRESH pineapple juice.

Make sure your skin is clean and oil-free or cream-free. Dip a cotton ball in the pineapple juice and place it on the spot. Leave it there for twenty minutes, then rinse with tepid water and pat dry. Do this every day and within a week the spots may fade away.

• Daily doses of vitamin E along with vitamin C have been known to decrease the accumulation of the pigment that causes the appearance of age spots. Check with your health professional for dosages that are appropriate for you.

Blemish Cleanser: Add two tablespoons of camomile (available at health food stores) to a pot of water. Bring it to a boil, then remove it from the burner. Take a large towel, put it over your head, and put your head over the steaming pot. *Be careful. Do not get too close to the hot pot* . . . just close enough for the herbal steam to clean out your pores for five to ten minutes. After the steaming, let the air dry your skin.

Boils: A boil is an infection of a gland or a hair follicle. There are several foods that can help draw out the infection. Apply one of the following—

• A crushed, top-layer cabbage leaf.

• Cut a small red onion in half, take out a little center section of one half, then place the centerless half over the boil.

• A slice of tomato that has been warmed.

• The inside of a ripe (brown speckled) banana peel.

When a boil opens, the gook is expelled, the pain disappears, and there's a hole in the skin. Add two tablespoons of fresh lemon juice to a cup of just-boiled water. Use the lemon water to clean and disinfect the area. Then put a sterile bandage on it.

Chapped Hands: Put two slices of lemon and two slices of orange in a wooden bowl (metal or plastic is a no-no). Heat half-and-half (cream and milk)—twice as much as you need to cover the lemon and orange slices—so that it's a little warmer than taking the chill out. Pour the heated half-and-half over the fruit, cover the bowl, and leave it like that for three hours. Then strain and gently massage the liquid into your hands. Allow it to dry on the skin—give it about fifteen minutes—then remove it with a wet washcloth and a little olive oil.

For coming up with this remedy that can change rough, chapped, dishpan hands to soft, silky ones, let's give a hand to Dallas's beauty expert, Paul Neinast.

Dead Skin Cleanser: Once a week, slough off dead skin particles with an abrasive. Take a quarter cup of stone-ground cornmeal and mix in enough water to made a thick paste. Using an upward and outward motion, gently scrub your face with the cornmeal. Then wash it off with tepid water and wipe dry with that same upward and outward motion.

Another method is to dip cotton pads in fresh pineapple juice and put them on your face. Leave them on for fifteen minutes, then rinse your face with tepid water. For this to be an extremely effective dead skin slougher, you must use *fresh* pineapple juice only.

Eczema: These folk remedies for eczema work from the inside out—

• Eat one tablespoon of blackstrap molasses daily.

• Eat one raw potato a day.

• Eat a few teaspoons of watercress each day.

• Have one teaspoon of raw sesame oil daily, but only if you check with your health professional first, and only if you figure it into your daily fat gram allowance. Cooking with it doesn't count; you must have it raw.

• If you have a juice extractor, make yourself a daily green drink using green vegetables (i.e., alfalfa sprouts, parsley, spinach, celery, lettuce).

• Drink an ounce of aloe vera juice after each meal. (If you have an aloe vera plant, apply the gel from the leaves to the affected area at least twice a day. If you don't have an aloe plant for your skin, use the same aloe juice you're drinking.)

An effective external treatment is to put the contents of two chaparral capsules into a pint of just-boiled water. Cover and let it stand until it's cool—at least ten minutes. Strain through a superfine strainer or through unbleached muslin. Dip a white washcloth in the chapparal tea and put it on the sore spots. Do it twice a day for fifteen minutes at a time.

Facials: Some facials will deep-clean the skin, nourish the skin, tone and tighten the skin, and stimulate circulation. For a facial to be effective, you should start with a clean face and neck.

Facial Conditioners: When honeydews are in season, mash the meat of the melon and smear it on your face and neck. After twenty minutes, rinse with cool water and pat dry.

Or, combine two tablespoons of light cream or plain yogurt with one teaspoon of raw honey. Smear it on your face using an upward and outward motion. After fifteen minutes, wash it off with tepid water and pat dry.

Facial for Sensitive Skin: Mix one tablespoon of sour cream with one tablespoon of wheat germ flour until it has a creamy consistency. Spread it on your face and neck and relax with it on for twenty minutes. Then rinse off with tepid water and pat dry. Do this at least once a week.

Facial for Dry Skin: Actress and beauty authority Arlene Dahl shared her favorite facial mask with us.

Beat two egg yolks and apply them to your clean face, forehead, and neck, carefully avoiding the sensitive area around your eyes. Leave it on for twenty minutes as you relax on a slant board with your feet about thirty degrees higher than your head. If you don't have a slant board, improvise. Do not talk while you are relaxing—the egg yolk can crack on your face and you don't want that to happen.

At the end of twenty minutes, gently wash your face with

lukewarm water and pat it dry. You should feel just great with your skin tightened and toned. Do this at least once a week.

Both of us met Arlene Dahl at a TV studio. The lights were as bright as could be and we stood right next to her. Not only is she gracious and lovely, she's truly beautiful! I don't know about you, but . . . Lydia, get out the egg yolks.

Oily Skin Facial: Use the same procedure as for dry skin (see above), but use egg *whites* instead of yolks.

Incidentally, Arlene Dahl told us that both of these facials were used by Cleopatra. Like most women at different stages of their lives, Cleo's skin must have changed from oily to dry.

Freckles: Forget removing freckles. We think the most you can hope for is making them lighter. If you're interested in that, then rub your freckles with slices of fresh, raw eggplant every day. That's known to lighten them. Or, rub fresh, crushed cranberries on your bespeckled skin. Do this on a daily basis, leaving it on for fifteen minutes. Rinse with cool water and pat dry.

If you're really determined to make light of your freckles, collect six ounces of urine in a jar, add a tablespoon of white vinegar and a pinch of salt. Cover the jar and twenty-four hours later, with a cotton ball, pat the solution on the freckles. After a half hour, rinse with cool water. Do this every day until the freckles fade, or until you begin to appreciate your charming natural adornment.

It is said that the more refined sugar you eat, the darker your freckles are going to be. This sounds like an old wives' tale. It isn't. It's based on scientific research. Conclusion: Eliminate refined sugar from your diet and watch your freckles fade.

Grimy Hands Cleanser: When your hands are downright dirty, use olive oil to clean off the grime, the grease, and the tar. Vigorously massage the olive oil into the hands, then wipe them with paper towels. For hard-to-get-out stains, you may have to oil your hands again, adding some sugar as an abrasive. To get the olive oil off your hands, rinse them with warm water and wipe them with some more paper towels.

Hives: Right now, out of every thousand people, eleven men and fourteen women have hives.

Thoroughly blend one ounce of white vinegar with three ounces of cornstarch and dab the hives with the mixture. It's an antiseptic; it stops itching, and it can dry up the hives.

Makeup Cleanser: Sesame oil or almond oil on a cotton ball will do a thorough job of taking off makeup, including waterproof mascara.

Moisturizers: Moisturizers do not nourish the skin with moisture—they cover the skin with a thin film that *holds in* the skin's moisture. Use a moisturizer after cleansing.

• Using a plant mister, spray your face thoroughly with spring water or distilled water. Then pat on a thin layer of sesame oil. The oil should prevent the water from quickly disappearing and your hungry dry skin will soak up moisture for hours. You may want to add a few drops of perfume to the sesame oil.

• Dallas beauty expert Paul Neinast of the Neinast Salon recommends green Thompson seedless grapes as a moisturizer. Cut each grape in half and gently crush it on your face and neck. Be sure to let the grape juice get at the corners of your mouth and around your eyes. According to Paul, it's great for getting rid of crow's feet and the tiny cracks around the edges of the mouth.

Leave it on for about twenty minutes and then wash it off with tepid water and pat dry.

Pimple Prevention . . . Sort Of: Pimples take 90 days to form. The second you feel or notice a pimple forming, put an ice cube on it and keep it there for 3 to 5 minutes. Do this a few times throughout the day, until there's no trace of the pimple.

Pore-Closer and Skin Tightener: In keeping with the grapes in the remedy above, Paul Neinast also recommends a champagne skin splash—like a man splashes after-shave lotion—to close pores and tighten loose, slightly sagging skin, especially beneath the eyes and around the throat.

Psoriasis: In our books and during most every public appearance, we make mention of the fact that we are reporting, not prescribing. This is no exception. We're reporting a fascinating observation made by Dr. Ronald N. Shore of Johns Hopkins.

Dr. Shore took a small skin sample from a psoriasis sufferer and covered the cut with a Band-Aid. Three weeks later, when the Band-Aid was removed, the skin under the *adhesive* portion of the Band-Aid had cleared completely. After conducting many experiments, Dr. Shore feels that, since psoriasis lesions cleared up totally in only a minority of patients, the adhesive would be more effective in conjunction with other therapies.

Dr. I. William Lane in his book, *Sharks Don't Get Cancer,* reports on the successful use of shark cartilage for psoriasis. "Experience is limited," says Dr. Lane, "but already indicates that the effective dosage level for psoriasis is 1 gram per 15 pounds of body weight taken for 60 to 90 days."

"Be aware," Dr. Lane cautions, "in this treatment, the itching and scales will be the first symptoms to disappear. Without the scales, the redness of the skin will appear to intensify since the large bed of capillary vessels will be more apparent. This capillary bed will also slowly disappear."

Look for unadulterated 100% pure shark cartilage such as Benefin or Cartilade. It's available at most health food stores, vitamin shops, and pharmacies, and it's costly, but if it works, it's worth it. And if it doesn't work, you'll know by the end of 90 days.

According to Dr. Ray Wunderlich Jr. children, athletes, and people with compromised circulation should be wary of prolonged usage. Be sure to check with your health professional before starting any self-help program.

• Drink an ounce of aloe vera juice after each meal. If you have an aloe vera plant, apply the gel from the leaves to the affected area at least twice a day. If you don't have an aloe plant for your skin, use the same aloe juice you're drinking.

• Studies show that substituting Omega-3 fish oils for other fats in your diet may help heal psoriasis. Check with your health professional to determine the right amount of fish oil for you.

• Burdock root (available at health food stores) has been known to help clear up severe cases of psoriasis. Prepare tea by bringing four cups of water to a boil. Add a heaping tablespoon of dried burdock root, cover, and let simmer on a very low flame for a half hour. Strain, then divide the liquid into two portions. Drink each portion on an empty stomach: one portion before breakfast and the other before dinner. Do this daily and watch for results within a few weeks.

• There seems to be a connection between psoriasis sufferers and an inability to digest gluten. Gluten is a protein found in grain. Try a gluten-free diet. That means no wheat, oats, barley, or rye. It doesn't mean bye-bye bread. Check your health food store for gluten-free baked products.

Rejuvenator for Dry and Aging Skin: Peel a peach, remove the pit, then mash the peach meat. Apply it to your freshly-washed face and neck. (It's good for hands, too.) Leave it on for 20 minutes, then rinse with cool water. It should restore the acid balance and regenerate tissue of dry, aging skin.

Skin Spoiler: If you don't want deep wrinkles around the eyes and lips long before Mother Nature intended them to be there, or if you dread the thought of looking in a mirror and seeing that your skin has a grayish-yellowish pallor and the texture of dry leather, then don't let a cigarette touch your lips. If you're already a smoker, stop—the quality of your complexion will improve.

Under-Eye Puffiness and Dark Circles: Prepare one big poultice or two smaller ones with a grated raw potato in unbleached muslin or layered cheesecloth. Place the poultice(s) over your closed eyes on your lids and under your eyes. Leave it on for twenty relaxing minutes. Wash with cool water and pat dry. Puff!—No puffiness.

To lighten the dark circles under your eyes, you have to repeat the above procedure every day and maybe get a little more sleep every night.

Wrinkles Away: Almond oil (available at health food stores) is said to soften the little lines around the eyes and mouth. Gently massage the oil on the problem areas twice a day.

Wrinkle Prevention: Don't be a pillow-puss. Sleeping with your face pressed into the pillow causes wrinkles. Train yourself to sleep on your back or on your side with your face off the pillow.

Give yourself regular wrinkle-prevention facials. Blend equal amounts of plain yogurt and brewer's yeast together until smooth. Spread it on your face and neck and leave it on for twenty minutes. Then rinse off with tepid water and pat dry. Do this twice a week.

Wrinkle Removers: Paul Neinast of Dallas's famous Neinast Salon says that if you follow this treatment in the morning and again in the evening wrinkles should begin to disappear within weeks and your skin can look years younger—

In a wooden bowl (metal or plastic is a no-no), put two slices of lemon. Heat half-and-half (enough to cover the lemon slices), so that it's a little warmer than taking the chill out. If your skin is oily, use four slices of lemon. If you have dry skin, use one slice of lemon and use twice as much half-and-half.

Pour the heated half-and-half over the lemon, cover the bowl, and leave like that for three hours. Then strain and gently massage the liquid into your face and neck, with your middle three fingertips, in circular upward and outward motions. Allow it to dry on the skin—give it about fifteen minutes—then remove it with a wet washcloth and a little olive oil.

To prepare for this next treatment, pin your hair out of the way and wash your face and neck with warm water. Next, with your fingers, spread a thin layer of raw honey on your face and neck. Leave it on for twenty minutes, then rinse with tepid water and pat dry.

Raw honey can do wonders for the skin—everything from clearing up blemishes, holding in moisture, and restoring weather-beaten skin to smoothing away wrinkles.

❧ SLEEP DISORDERS ❧

Sound sleep is one of the foundations of good health. To ensure a good night's sleep and a gentle awakening, arrange your bedroom so that it has a calming influence on you.

• Paint the walls a soft, quiet color—blue, pink, or green. It can make a big difference in your night's sleep, even though your eyes are closed.

• Make sure that the things you see right before falling asleep do not stimulate your nervous system, or aggravate you in any way. In other words, you don't want a desk near your bed, reminding you of all the work you have to do. You don't want to see the folder with all your unpaid bills calling out, "Overdue! Overdue!"

• Aside from a good reading light next to or over your bed, have soft, flattering lighting in the bedroom, making it feel cozy and warm.

• End the day and start your night's sleep with comforting, positive, and optimistic thoughts. (See the *Affirmation* at the end of this chapter.)

How much sleep is enough? According to research done at the Henry Ford Hospital in Detroit, chances are you need more sleep than you're getting. Experiment by going to sleep a half hour earlier than usual each night for a week. If you don't feel more alert and energetic, go to sleep an hour earlier the second week.

Be sure you go to sleep at an earlier hour at night, rather than sleeping an hour later in the morning. If you sleep later in the A.M., the morning metabolic increases in body temperature and hormones may be depressed and can result in sluggishness and lethargy.

For occasional insomnia, try these natural remedies:

• Open your mouth and remember how it feels to yawn. Bring on a yawn . . . and another one . . . and another. Yawning makes you feel sleepy, and chances are, you'll be asleep before your yawning jag ends.

• Chop a yellow onion in chunks and place the chunks in a jar with a cover. Place the jar on your night table. Once you're in bed and having trouble falling asleep, uncover the jar and take a deep whiff of the onion. Re-cover the jar, lie back, and think lovely thoughts. You should be asleep within fifteen minutes.

• Use all-cotton bed sheets. According to Debra Lynn Dadd, author of *Nontoxic, Natural, and Earthwise* (Jeremy P. Tarcher Inc., 1990), polyester-cotton sheets are coated with formaldehyde, a substance known to cause insomnia.

• Having a hard time falling asleep? The answer may be in your kitchen sink. In certain folkloric circles, it is believed that dirty dishes left undone can cause insomnia.

• Eat pumpkin—as a side dish or as a dessert—and your insomnia may be no more than a dream.

• The classic insomnia folk remedy is a pillow made of hops. Have you ever smelled hops? It's so vile, I think you fall asleep just to escape the smell.

We found something a lot more pleasant that's said to be just as effective. It's celery seeds. Stuff a little pillow with them and sleep on it.

• Once you're in bed and relaxed, take seven deep breaths—inhale to the count of seven; exhale to the count of seven. Wait three minutes, then take seven deep breaths again. Wait another three minutes and then take another seven deep breaths, that is, if you're not already asleep.

• Have a cup of herbal slumber-inspiring tea: camomile, dill, heather, anise, a nephew (just testing to see if you're asleep yet), peppermint, or rosemary.

Nightmares: The average adult has at least one nightmare a year. One in 500 people has nightmares once a week. About five percent of the adult population has nightmares even more often than once a week.

We got this remedy from a reputable radio host in Rhode Island. Take a smelly sock—*your* smelly sock—wrap the instep of the sock around your throat, and sleep that way. It will not only cure a sore throat, it will prevent nightmares.

Gem Therapy for Occasional Insomnia and Nightmares: Hold a piece of amethyst in your hand to help you fall asleep. Place a piece of amethyst in your pillowcase to prevent nightmares.

Talking While Asleep: Take hold of the big toe of a person who's talking in his sleep and he'll tell you anything you want to know. This remedy came to us from the hills of South Dakota . . . or was it from a California divorce lawyer?

Putting a Stop to Snoring: Anthony Burgess said, "Laugh and the world laughs with you, snore and you sleep alone." To prevent that from happening, stop drinking and stop smoking and, chances are, you'll stop snoring. Alcohol and cigarettes cause the swelling of tissues that cause snoring.

Have you ever heard a person with a whiplash injury snore? They don't. Well, not if they sleep with a cervical collar around their neck. The collar prevents the chin from resting on the chest—a position that partially closes the windpipe and causes snoring. When you wear the collar, the chin stays up and the windpipe stays open.

If someone else is snoring, make a clacking noise with your tongue, the noise you make to imitate the clippity-clop of a horse. It works. It will either make the snorer stop snoring, or it will awaken the snorer, in which case he or she will stop snoring.

♪ **Affirmation:** Repeat this affirmation at bedtime, over and over until you fall asleep—

I let go of all the pressures of the day in exchange for a good night's sleep. I feel in harmony with the universe, and secure with myself.

REFERRAL

For informative brochures and referrals to regional sleep disorder centers, write to:

National Sleep Foundation
1367 Connecticut Avenue, N.W. Suite 200
Washington, DC 20036

SMOKING

I used to smoke, but I stopped
because I didn't want to be dependent on anything . . .
I can't let a little cigarette run my body.

—DIANA ROSS

Keep in mind that quitting smoking *now* greatly reduces serious risk to your health.

We're sure you already know a dozen of the most important reasons to stop smoking. Here are several you may not know—

• Smokers suffer from heartburn more often than nonsmokers, and also more indigestion, ulcers, and constipation.

• Smokers suffer from insomnia more often than nonsmokers.

• Since smoking decreases the flow of blood to the extremities, smokers tend to have cold hands and feet.

• Within three months of being nicotine-free, your circulation improves and lung function increases up to thirty percent.

• Throat dryness . . . smoking is the main cause.

• A smoker's complexion is generally dryer, more leathery looking, and the skin tone is drabber than nonsmokers'.

• A smoker is more likely to have more wrinkles around the eyes and lips than nonsmokers.

• If a smoker has a face lift, the blood vessels can constrict and affect the healing process.

• Men who smoke have a lower sperm count, less sperm mobility, and more abnormal sperm than nonsmoking men.

• Women who smoke have a higher percentage of miscarriages than nonsmoking women.

• After seventy-two hours without a cigarette, your bronchial tubes relax, making breathing easier.

- Stop smoking for at least five years and the risk of having a stroke will drop to just about the same chance as a non-smoker's.

- If you smoke near a tomato plant, the tobacco can give the tomatoes a virus that can kill them.

EBBING OFF CIGARETTES

Mix a half-teaspoon of cream of tartar (available in supermarket baking and/or spice sections) into eight ounces of orange juice and drink it before bedtime. The cream of tartar helps clear the nicotine out of your system.

Each cigarette you smoke robs your body of about twenty-five milligrams of vitamin C. The orange juice will help replace that vitamin C.

Once you've made up your mind to stop smoking and start this regimen, be consistent! Take the drink every night without fail. Then, the following day, when you reach for a cigarette, you may think twice about it. You may even be able to decide not to have that cigarette.

By reducing the number of cigarettes you have each day, you should be able to ebb off them completely and painlessly by the end of a month, if not sooner.

Make it easier *not* to smoke than to light up. These suggestions can help—

- As you're ebbing off, every time you buy a pack of cigarettes, change brands to ones that are less appealing to you. It will reduce the pleasure of smoking and it can affect your blood chemistry reaction, making it less torturous for you to break the habit.

- Do not buy cartons of cigarettes; buy one pack at a time, and only after you've finished a pack.

- Each day, wait an hour longer than the prior day before lighting your first cigarette.

- When you have a real craving for a cigarette, tell yourself you can have the cigarette in about five minutes; meanwhile, do something absorbing, something that takes your total concentration to do.

• Figure out your favorite times and situations for smoking and avoid them. For instance, if you always smoke while you're driving a car, take public transportation until you've kicked the habit.

• It's a good idea to hang out in places where smoking is prohibited and to hang out with people who don't smoke and mind if you do.

CIGARETTE SUBSTITUTES

Here are foods you can eat and things you can do to help resist the temptation to smoke—

• Instead of reaching for a cigarette, reach for a handful of raw, shelled sunflower seeds. They provide the same psychological boost you get from cigarettes and the nerve-calming effect of tobacco. Sunflower seeds also help nourish the nervous system. They're a great cigarette substitute!

• Take a tiny piece of fresh ginger root. It's strong and burns. It's that burning quality that makes it a good substitute for cigarettes. Unlike smoking a cigarette, ginger will make your mouth feel clean and refreshed.

• Juice a fresh radish by grating it or by putting it in a food processor and then squeezing the grated pulp through cheesecloth. Add honey to taste and drink the juice.

• Suck on a clove. It isn't fun to do, but it does lessen your desire for a cigarette.

• Quell the urge to light up by pressing the acupressure point in the middle of the breastbone directly between your two nipples. Press it three times in a row, for twelve seconds each time.

• There's thought to be a strong connection between acidic body chemistry and a craving for nicotine. If you decrease the acidic foods you eat and increase the alkalinic foods, you can cut down on your nicotine craving. Some alkalinizing foods are apples, berries, raisins, sweet potatoes, carrots, celery, mushrooms, onions, peas, lima beans, and almonds.

• At least once a day, instead of taking a cigarette or any of these substitute foods or drinks, resist the craving by taking ten slow, deep breaths of air. Don't be surprised if the deep breaths leave you completely satisfied.

• A few cups of slippery elm bark tea a day can help submerge the urge to smoke. You may want to alternate with oatstraw tea, marjoram tea, and magnolia bark tea—all available at most health food stores.

• To replace the physicality of a cigarette in your hand, you can hold a pen or pencil. If you really want something to play with, twist a paper clip, or invest in Chinese exercise balls (available at some Asian shops, health food stores, and through New Age catalogs listed in RESOURCES).

• Playing with a yo-yo can help divert your attention and relieve the stress of withdrawal. See Referrals for a catalog that advertises the wonderful Yomega Yo-Yo With A Brain.

♫ **Affirmation:** Repeat this affirmation seven times, starting first thing in the morning, every time you eat, drink, or do something *instead* of smoking a cigarette, and last thing at night.
I'm proud of the choices I make. My reward is good health and joy.

We greatly respect you for wanting to stop smoking and we send every good wish for your success.

When you've accomplished your goal, we would love to hear about it. If you want to share with us your triumph over that nasty habit, please write to us at P. O. Box 416, Ansonia Station, NYC 10023.

REFERRALS

Yo-Yo With A Brain   Free catalog
Yomega Corporation
1058 Pleasant Street

P.O. Box 4146
Fall River, MA 02723-0402
508/672-7399

Once you've quit smoking and want to join an organization that protects the rights of the nonsmoking majority by legal action and education on the hazards of smoking, write to:

ASH (Action on Smoking and Health)
2013 H Street, N.W. Suite B
Washington, DC 20006

SORE THROAT

This mild inflammation can lower your resistance and leave you vulnerable to other ailments that attack when resistances are lowered. Let's just nip this sore throat in the bud.

Caution: If your sore throat isn't gone after three days, see a health professional and be tested for strep throat.

Classic Sore Throat Remedy #1: Honey and lemon was a standard in our house. Mom would squeeze the juice of a lemon into a big mug of just-boiled water and add enough honey—one to three tablespoons—to make it delicious.

Or, in another version, mix a tablespoon of honey with the juice of a lemon—no water. Have it either way every couple of hours.

Classic Sore Throat Remedy #2: Mix two teaspoons of apple cider vinegar in a glass of warm water. Take a mouthful, gargle with it, and spit it out, then swallow a mouthful; gargle a mouthful, spit it out, and swallow a mouthful; gargle a mouthful—notice a pattern forming? Do this until there's no liquid left in the glass. Repeat the process once an hour. By the third or fourth hour, the sore throat is usually gone. (This remedy works for us every time.)

Classic Sore Throat Remedy #3: Dissolve a heaping teaspoon of salt (kosher salt is preferred; table salt will do) in a glass of warm water and gargle with it.

Now that we've reviewed the "classics," here is a variety of other remedies, ranging from the familiar to the they-must-work-or-why-would-they-include-them-in-the-book?

• Eat a few slices of fresh pineapple. A grapefruit can be effective, too, and so is drinking a glass of grapefruit juice.

• Throughout the day, drink horehound tea (available at health food stores). Simply steep a teaspoon of the herb in a cup of just-boiled water, and as soon as it's cool, strain and drink.

• Try this bartender's remedy. Instead of sucking candy to soothe your throat, suck on an olive. Remove the pit and keep the meat of the olive in your mouth until you finally chew it and swallow it. Then take another olive.

• Because of limited space, we can't reprint letters from people who graciously share their remedies with us. Of course there's always an exception and this is it:

> *Girls:*
> Here's a home remedy I used sixty-five years ago that is as amusing as it is effective. Don't ask me why it works, but it did when I was ten, and later when my daughters were about the same age.
> For a sore throat, when you retire, wrap your neck in a dirty sock. The dirtier the better.
> I reasoned it was the warmth, but a towel doesn't work; the sock does! No kidding!!
>
> *"Phewers" truly,*
> *Selwyn P. Miles*

Helpful hint to everyone who uses this remedy: Boil the soiled socks with a few lemon slices and they'll get sparkling white again.

Prevention: Bacteria can live on your toothbrush and reinfect you. As soon as your sore throat is completely gone, get a new toothbrush.

Acupressure: Massage deep into the weblike area between the thumb and the index finger. It can help relieve the rawness of an inflamed throat.

Aromatherapy: Essential pine oil has antiseptic properties. Add a couple of drops of the oil to a pot of just-boiled water and carefully inhale the vapor. Throughout the day, reheat the water with the pine oil and inhale.

♪ **Affirmation:** Whenever you look at a watch or clock, it's "time" to blow your own horn by repeating this affirmation at least fifteen times—

I am the best there is! I shout my praises loud and clear.

STREP THROAT

Strep throat should not be taken lightly. It can lead to serious repercussions if not treated properly. Proceed with professional medical supervision.

If you have a dog or cat and you get strep throat more often than once in a blue moon, you may be catching the streptococci from the animal. Get the vet to check the pet. When your pet is free of the bacteria, you probably will be, too.

Strep Throat Remedy: Every hour, take three alfalfa tablets and every third hour add 100 mgs of vitamin C. Start this regimen in the morning and stop at bedtime. If you're not all better the next morning, do it for another day. Remember . . . professional medical supervision, please.

LARYNGITIS

Do you cradle the receiver between your shoulder and neck while you talk on the telephone? If that's what you do, you may be straining your larynx in order to produce sounds when your head is tilted. If that's what's causing your laryngitis, hang up the phone and go get yourself one of those headsets.

Though you may not figure out what caused your laryngitis, you'll soon be able to tell everyone about your speedy recovery if you follow these suggestions:

• Stay away from cold drinks. Cold fluids can make the problem worse. It's best to drink warm—not hot—water and other liquids . . . and lots of it.

• Since you want to keep the larynx moist, alcoholic beverages—even the so-called *medicinal mixtures*—are a no-no. They just dry out the larynx.

• Stay away from any kind of mint or mentholated drinks or cough drops. They can dry out your vocal cords.

• Do not gargle. Your vocal cords do not need the stress that gargling causes.

• Do not whisper. Whispering also stresses the vocal cords. In fact, shut up! For a day or two, write instead of talk.

LARYNGITIS REMEDIES

• Slippery elm bark (available at health food stores) can be made into a tea by following the directions on the box. Drink three or four cups a day for a soothing glaze on the vocal cords and relief from the pain of an abused throat.

• Remove the shells of a few uncooked chestnuts and chew them like you would chew gum. It's said to be helpful in curing laryngitis.

• Prepare strong sage tea by using a heaping teaspoon of the herb in a cup of just-boiled water. Let it steep for ten minutes, strain, and drink. Sage will not only help heal the laryngitis, it will also strengthen your voice. Drink three cups a day until your voice is back to normal.

Attempting to remove a splinter with tweezers may make the problem worse. The tweezers may push the splinter deeper into the skin, or break off the splinter and leave part of it embedded beneath the skin. Save the tweezers for your eyebrows, and consider the simple, safer splinter-removing methods below.

Easy-to-Remove Splinter Remedy: This is one of those "Why didn't I think of it?" remedies. Take a piece of tape—Scotch or adhesive—and put it on the splinter. It will also work with a thin layer of school-type white glue spread on the splintered area. Try to figure out the direction in which the splinter is facing so that you can yank off the tape or the glob of glue accordingly. If it doesn't work the first time, give it a second or third try.

Hard-to-Remove Splinter Remedy: Wrap a strip of raw bacon around the area with the splinter and cover the bacon with a piece of cloth. Keep on overnight and in the morning; when you remove the bacon, chances are, you will also remove the splinter.

Hardest-to-Remove Splinter Remedy: Take a teaspoon of ground fenugreek (available at most health food stores) and add enough water to make a paste of it. Place it on the sore area and wrap gauze around it. Keep it on overnight. In the morning, when you clear away the fenugreek, the splinter should have surfaced and you can scrape it or tape it off. (See the first splinter "tape" remedy above.)

STIFF NECK

Pillow Talk: Foam rubber pillows may be at the bottom of a lot of neck problems. Because of the foam's bounciness, there may be a strain to keep the head in place. Try sleeping on a nonfoam pillow for at least a week and see if the stiff neck is gone.

The Radish Remedy: Prepare a poultice out of grated radishes. Obviously, we can't tell you how many radishes to use; it depends on the size of the radishes and the size of your neck area. Be sure the poultice is long enough to go around your neck and wide enough to dip down and rest on your back and shoulders. To keep the radishes' heat in, put plastic film around the poultice and leave it on for a half hour. During that half hour, you might want to repeat the affirmation (below) over and over. It couldn't hurt. Humor us, okay?

Acupressure: Vigorously massage the area a drop below the base of the little toe. Massage for at least five minutes and you should feel less pain and stiffness in your neck. Ideal, is to get someone to massage both feet at the same time. Even though your neck will feel better after the first massage, continue massaging three times a day for a couple of days.

♪ Affirmation: Repeat this affirmation at least ten times, first thing in the morning and each time you nod your head and feel the stiffness—

I stir up the gifts within me and use them to face all challenges. I am a real winner.

STRESS, TENSION, ANXIETY, NERVOUSNESS, AND PANIC

Some great minds of our time have written about stress, tension, and anxiety. When you read what they have to say, it doesn't seem to sound so bad after all. In fact, reading these things actually calmed me down, making me feel a whole lot better.

According to Felix Morley, "From tension . . . all human progress springs."

"It is well to remind ourselves," says Dr. Rollo May, "anxiety signifies a conflict, and so long as a conflict is going on, a constructive solution is possible."

Dr. Stanley J. Sarnoff of the National Institute of Health, said, "The process of living is the process of reacting to stress."

On coping with stress, this is how Dr. Robert S. Eliot, cardiology professor at the University of Nebraska, sums it up: "Rule Number 1 is, don't sweat the small stuff. Rule Number 2 is, it's all small stuff. And if you can't fight and you can't flee, flow."

Here are some suggestions for flowing—

Daily Unwind: Find a convenient, comfortable place to take a one-hour vacation every single day. When you wake up in the morning, make an appointment with yourself, name a specific time, and keep to it. During that hour, do whatever relaxes you. Read, watch TV, do a crossword puzzle, knit, listen to music (more about that a little later)—whatever gives you pleasure.

Unburden Yourself: Writer Garson Kanin said, "There are thousands of causes for stress, and one antidote to stress is self-expression. That's what happens to me every day. My thoughts get off my chest, down my sleeves and onto my pad."

Get it off *your* chest and onto a pad. Keep a diary. You may want to spend ten minutes of your daily vacation (see remedy above) to let it all out on paper.

Portable Anti-Stress Machine: Stress is always with us—during rush-hour traffic, while trying to find a public phone that works, being told the computer is down after waiting on line at the bank.

What we need, according to Stuart F. Crump, Jr., is an anti-stress machine that's as portable as our problems. And he has one. It's a yo-yo. Actually, Stuart, also known as "Professor Yo-Yo," has 500 of them. He says that yo-yoing is an excellent way to cope with stress throughout the day, wherever you are. Most of us did it as children, and once you know how, you never forget.

So start playing with a yo-yo and you can have the world on a string!

Music Hath Charms to Soothe: Let go of tension and anxiety by listening to calming music. There is a big selection of tapes in health food stores. Select instrumentals—no vocalists—and stick with slow, regular rhythms that feature piano and string instruments—harp, guitar, violin, and cello. Avoid brass instruments. (See "Healing Music" in the Well-Being Chapter.)

Calm-Down Tea: The classic folk remedy to calm the nerves and help you relax is camomile tea (available at health food stores). Steep a teaspoon of the herb in a cup of just-boiled water. After five minutes, strain and sip slowly.

Hot vs. Cold: Some say that a cold bath or shower is invigorating and can convert your nervous tension into creative energy. Others think a hot bath or shower improves circulation and encourages your body to relax. Whatever works for you.

Natural Tranquilizer: When you need to be more tranquil, prepare a cup of catnip tea (available at health food stores) by steeping a heaping teaspoon of catnip in a cup of just-boiled water. After five minutes, strain and drink. If you have a cat, be sure to put the catnip away in a secure place, or your feline will make a beeline for it.

Or, try calming your jittery nerves with celery juice. If you don't have a juice extractor, find a health food store that has a juice bar and order celery juice either straight or with some carrot juice mixed in.

Vitamin Therapy: Experts agree, taking a super B-complex vitamin daily may reduce feelings of tension and anxiety.

Shall We Tense: This easy-to-do exercise will take the stress right out of your body in no time. If possible, lie down on the floor with your eyes closed. If that's impractical, sit with your eyes closed. Make a fist with both hands and tense the muscles in your fingers, wrists, and forearms. Stay that way for five seconds, then release the tension, letting it fall away from your fingers, wrists, and forearms. Continue the tensing/relaxing process with your shoulders, neck and face, your legs, feet, and toes. Notice the uncomfortable feeling when you tense up; then fully enjoy the experience of relaxing.

If you practice this at least once a day, you'll soon be able to do it quickly and effectively whenever you need to de-stress.

Reach for Sesame: When something stressful happens suddenly, the blood calcium level can drop, making the situation seem worse. Reach for a handful of sesame seeds, or any other food rich in calcium. It can help you get through an unanticipated emotional upheaval.

PANIC ATTACKS

When that sudden wave of terror strikes, you know exactly what it is . . . it's a panic attack. Since you know what it is, there's no need to panic. It's a temporary horror that lasts a matter of minutes. The less panicky you get, the quicker it will pass.

The second it starts, say to yourself, "This is a panic attack and it will be over very soon. Now I'll relax and start my controlled breathing exercise."

To the count of five, take a deep breath in through your nostrils, hold it for another count of five, then breathe out through your mouth to the count of ten. Keep concentrating on the five-five-ten breathing process and, before long, that panicky feeling will be gone.

Have you seen a health professional about your panic attacks? If you have and you're both convinced that the attacks are not caused by a physical problem like hypoglycemia or PMS, but by stress, consider these suggestions—

• Confront fearful situations instead of worrying about them.

• Don't sit around second-guessing every possible scenario. Instead, go directly to the source—call the person who has the answer(s) you need.

• Exercise daily, even if it's just taking a brisk walk for a half hour.

• Eat a well-balanced diet . . . but that's an old story. Also, stay away from soda, caffeine, and anything with sugar. No one said it's going to be easy.

• Be kind to your sensitive soul. That means don't read, watch, or listen to bad news. When you do watch TV, listen to the radio, go to a movie, or read, choose lighthearted things . . . uppers. Avoid TV's two-hour disease-of-the-month movie. Opt for *laughs* over *lumps; funny* instead of *fatal; joy-inspiring* rather than *panic-provoking*.

NERVE-RACKING SITUATIONS

We didn't know what the heading should be for these remedies, but all we had to do was mention some examples—making a speech, asking for a raise, going for a job interview—and we thought of the three words that sum it up best: Nerve-Racking Situations.

• If you have to make a presentation or do some kind of public speaking, limit your intake of caffeine and alcoholic beverages for at least twelve hours before your event. Do not drink milk or ice cold drinks two hours prior to your performance.

• The effect of aromatherapy on the psyche is potent and immediate. So, right before "showtime," take a couple of whiffs of black pepper. No, not *ground* black pepper. That'll make you sneeze. There are aromatherapy inhalers available at most health food stores and one of the scents is black pepper. A few whiffs can boost confidence and amplify courage.

• Think of a time you did something that was super. Re-live the feeling you felt, knowing you were wonderful and appreciated. Remember that feeling and re-create it as you present yourself.

Reflexology: Put your palms together against your chest as though you're praying. Intertwine your fingers and stay that way for about five minutes, until your entire body feels relaxed. Be sure your feet are flat on the floor and your shoulders are down. Closing your eyes may make you feel even more relaxed.

Gem Therapy: Rhodochrosite is the stone for relieving stress and anxiety. Wear it, carry it, stomp on it, throw it through a plate glass window. Only kidding. Just wear it or carry it.

Meditation: Choose a word that has a calming and uplifting influence on you. If you can think of one that ends with an "m" sound or an "n" sound, do so. Here are some examples: charm, fun, home, tame, win.

Sit in a comfortable chair, eyes closed and body relaxed. Say that word to yourself over and over each time you exhale. If your mind drifts, the second you realize it, go back to the word, and say it over and over while exhaling. Do this every day for fifteen minutes. If you find it a pleasant and beneficial experience, you may want to meditate twice a day.

This form of meditating can make a tremendous difference in your central nervous system. It can also lower your blood pressure and slow down your heart rate.

Visualization: When you feel tension building, or if you're already stressed out, take ten minutes to re-condition your transmission with this simple visualization exercise.

Sit in a comfortable chair and close your eyes. Breathe out all the air in your lungs, then slowly breathe in. As you exhale, visualize a huge theater marquee with bright lights flashing the number "3" three times. Take another slow, deep breath, and as you exhale, visualize the number "2" flashing three times. Take one more deep breath, slowly, and when you exhale, see the number "1" flashing three times.

Now that you're relaxed, picture paradise on earth. What is or would be your favorite place in the whole wide world? The beach? A cabin in the mountains? A field of flowers? Imagine yourself being there—wherever you'd be happiest. Feel free to thoroughly enjoy the visit for a few minutes.

When you're ready to return to the here-and-now, slowly count from one to three. Open your eyes, stretch, and notice how refreshed you feel.

That little getaway gives you the chance to let go of stress, allowing the body's healing energy to take over.

REFERRALS

For a wide selection of pure essence inhalers, call, write, or fax for a brochure or to place an order:

Nature's Apothecary
6350 Gunpark Drive Suite 500
Boulder, CO 80301
800/999-7422
Fax: 303/581-9883

Yo-Yo With A Brain   Free catalog
Yomega Corporation
1058 Pleasant Street
P.O. Box 4146
Fall River, MA 02723-0402
508/672-7399

For a free copy of Professor Yo-Yo's newsletter, call or send a stamped, self-addressed envelope to:

Yo-Yo Times
P.O. Box 1519—Dep't JL
Herndon, VA 22070
800/YO-YO MAN

SUNBURN

Do you know that you can actually get sunburned while swimming under water? You can also get a sunburn from the reflected rays of the sand, the water, and even cement. And it doesn't have to be a sunny day. You can get a severe sunburn on foggy and hazy days.

When you get a sunburn, you shed the top layer of *burned* skin and the new top layer of skin is then extremely sensitive to the sun. It takes three months for your skin to be the same as it was before the sunburn.

What we're getting at with all this information is that you must take precautions. Always use a sunscreen, wear a hat with a brim, wear sunglasses and, above all, use common sense if you want to save your skin—literally.

If you're careless enough to go out without proper protection, here are some remedies to help heal your sunburned skin—

• As soon as possible, take a cold shower. You know how you run cold water on pasta to stop the cooking process? Yup! The cold water stops the skin from continuing to burn.

Next, mix equal amounts of baking soda and cornstarch, depending on how much skin got sunburned, then add enough water to make a paste. Apply it to the affected areas.

If a lot of you is sunburned, pour cornstarch and baking soda into a cool bath and relax in it a while. When you get out, forget the towel—just dry off naturally with the cornstarch and soda on your skin.

• Apply aloe vera gel directly on the sunburned areas. Aloe vera gel is available at health food stores, or you can buy an aloe plant and squeeze the gel out of the leaves yourself.

Buying an aloe is like buying a pharmacy. There are close to one hundred medical uses for this easy-to-grow succulent.

• Mix equal amounts of apple cider vinegar and water. Gently sponge the mixture on the sunburned skin. It helps restore the acid mantle.

• Smear the sunburned areas with wheat germ oil, and don't be surprised if the red turns tan as it helps heal the skin.

• Ron Hamilton of Great American Natural Products shared his soothing sunburn remedy with us.

In a blender, put one peeled cucumber, one-half cup of oatmeal, one teaspoon of dried comfrey or slippery elm (either is optional), and one-half cup of yogurt. Blend well, then apply directly on the sunburned areas. It should give you quick relief as it takes out the pain and the redness.

• At the Neinast Salon in Dallas, Texas, beauty expert Paul Neinast treats sunburned faces by soaking slices of tomato in buttermilk for about ten minutes and applying the slices to the face. They relieve the pain, draw out the heat, and close the pores all at the same time.

For Peeling Skin: Mash the meat of a ripe papaya and put it on the peeling skin. Papaya, with all its wonderful enzymes, helps tone the skin while it removes dead cells. Keep on for a half hour, then rinse it off with cool water.

For Sunburned Eyes: Grate a raw potato and wrap it in cheesecloth. Put this potato poultice on your closed eyes and let it stay there, while you relax, for at least a half hour. Oh—and promise yourself that you'll never let this happen again.

Or, moisten a couple of tea bags under the cold water faucet and put them on your eyelids. Let them stay there for at least a half hour. If the tea bags dry up in that time, wet them again and reapply them.

Fail-Safe Overall Sunburn Prevention: The sun is strongest between 10 A.M. and 2 P.M. (standard time). If you go out *before* 9 A.M. or *after* 5 P.M., when the sunburn rays are screened out by the atmosphere, and stay in the rest of the day, you'll never run the risk of getting a sunburn.

𝒮 **Affirmation:** While treating the problem with any of the above remedies, repeat this affirmation at least fifteen times an hour until the heat is out of the sunburned skin—

I am calm. I have peace of mind. There's happiness in my heart.

TEETH, GUMS, AND MOUTH

Julius Caesar, Hannibal, and Napoleon had something unique in common. Each was born with a tooth in his mouth. Can you imagine?—three months old and already a plaque problem. The odds of a baby being born with a tooth showing are one in two thousand. Those are statistics that we have no control over.

A full set of teeth consists of thirty-two teeth. The average working adult has about twenty-four teeth. And by the time that adult is sixty-five, (s)he is down to an average of fourteen teeth. More than half of all people over the age of seventeen are in the early stages of some type of gum disease. These are statistics we *do* have control over with proper tooth and gum care.

Children should have a dental checkup every six months; adults should see their dentist once a year. Meanwhile, here are suggestions until you get to the dentist (these are not meant to *replace* the dentist)—

TOOTHACHE RELIEF

To ease the pain of a toothache while waiting for the dentist's appointment, you may want to try one of these—

• Dip a cotton ball in fresh lime juice and put it on your aching tooth.

• Rub cinnamon oil on the painful area.

• Take a little chunk of peanut butter, put mustard or mustard powder on it, and place it, mustard-side down, on the sore tooth. The peanut butter is used to hold the mustard in place.

- When you have a toothache and swollen gums, crush a half-cup of sesame seeds and put it in a small pot with a cup of water. Boil it until you have about a half-cup of water. Then strain out the seeds and use the liquid as a mouthwash to relieve the pain and swelling.

- Squeeze the gel from the leaf of an aloe vera plant directly on the tooth. Keep doing that until the pain completely disappears, the plant disappears, or it's time for your dentist appointment.

- This unusual remedy is said to work with horseradish or with garlic. Grate a two-ounce piece of fresh horseradish, wrap each ounce in two unbleached pieces of muslin or cheesecloth, and put them in the bend of each arm. If you prefer garlic, peel and mince two cloves and . . . you know the rest.

   Actually, placing a piece of horseradish or garlic directly on the problem tooth can relieve the pain.

- Steep a heaping teaspoon of yarrow in a few ounces of just-boiled water. After a minute, strain out the liquid and with the remaining moist herb make a tiny poultice in a little piece of cheesecloth to put on your sore tooth.

MINIMIZE DENTAL WORK PAIN AND PROMOTE HEALING

The bad news is that you need dental work. The good news is, here are several things you can do to help reduce the pain and speed up the healing—

- Starting a week before the dentist's first treatment, take ten mgs vitamin B-1 (thiamine) daily.

- Starting two weeks before dental work, eat a cup or two of pineapple canned in its own juice daily, and drink a cup of unsweetened pineapple juice as well. Following your dental appointment, drink a cup or two of pineapple juice. This should help reduce the discomfort that usually follows dental work, particularly oral surgery.

- After extensive dental work or oral surgery, mix one teaspoon of liquid chlorophyll in a half-cup of water and gently swish it around your mouth. Swallow it or spit it out—the choice is yours. Do this three-minute process a half-dozen times a day.

• After a treatment, relieve the discomfort by rubbing peppermint oil on the gums, covering the area with the teeth on which the work was done. You may have to do this every few hours until the pain stops recurring.

PREVENT TOOTH DECAY

This information falls into the you're-not-born-knowing-this category . . . perhaps it's the why-didn't-you-tell-me-sooner category . . . then again, maybe it's the I-wish-I-didn't-know/ignorance-is-bliss category.

• Whatever you do, don't suck a lemon . . . or any other citrus fruit. They can gradually dissolve calcium from your teeth. After eating an orange, grapefruit, lemon, or tangerine, or after drinking any kind of citrus drink, rinse your mouth with water . . . thoroughly.

• Tooth enamel loses minerals and grows softer within five minutes of drinking cola.

• The *Journal of the American Dental Association* published the results of a study that says raisins stick to your teeth and, therefore, cause more cavities than all other standard snacks, including caramel, fudge, chocolate, and cookies. So, after eating raisins, be sure to brush your teeth to prevent cavities.

PREVENT PLAQUE FORMATION

The bacteria and food particles in your mouth form plaque. Plaque, if not brushed away regularly, builds up and causes cavities, gum problems, and bad breath. Aside from diligent brushing and flossing, here are some plaque repellents to drink and/or eat after meals—

• Black cherry juice
• Raw apple

- Strawberries

- Aged cheeses, especially after eating sugary food or drinking cola—the cheese must be aged—cheddar, Swiss, Monterey Jack are best—eating a half-ounce of the cheese is adequate.

- Coffee or tea

- Chewing sugarless gum for at least ten minutes after you've eaten will produce saliva that will counterbalance the acid in the plaque. According to researchers at the Indiana University School of Dentistry, the potential for tooth decay decreased by an average seventy-two percent when patients chewed gum after eating.

TEETH CLENCHING AND GRINDING (BRUXISM)

When Kenneth R. Goljan, D.D.S., started practicing dentistry, teeth clenching and grinding were problems for elderly patients. As the years went on, the patients with the problem became younger and younger. Now, over twenty-eight years later, Dr. Goljan in Tulsa, Oklahoma, treats pre-teens who are clenching and grinding their teeth.

The doctor feels this problem relates to today's pressure-packed lifestyle which includes increased and immediate media coverage, compounding our self-generated stress.

Now that we know what may cause bruxism, here is Dr. Goljan's "Seven-by-Seven" system to help put an end to the problem. This system has been tested, fine-tuned, and used successfully on many people for close to ten years. Follow it exactly as it's written here.

In your own comfortable words, write down the answers to these four questions—keep the answers simple:

1. What is the problem? (Sample answer: "Clenching and grinding my teeth is bad for me.")
2. Why is it a problem? (Sample answer: "It causes me pain and makes me unhappy.")

3. What are you going to do about the problem? (Sample answer: "I will not clench and grind my teeth anymore.")

4. Why do you want to do something about the problem? (Sample answer: "This will make the pain disappear and I will be happier.")

Study your four phrases; analyze them, and when you're sure there aren't any hidden or double meanings that your subconscious can choose and act on, then memorize them. This is where the "Seven-by-Seven" comes in. You are to say your four answers seven times in a row, seven times a day. According to Dr. Goljan, the best times to do it are our landmark times: (1) breakfast, (2) between breakfast and lunch, (3) lunch, (4) between lunch and dinner, (5) dinner, (6) between dinner and bedtime, (7) bedtime.

The ideal situation is for you to be in a comfortable environment and to say the words out loud, with feeling. If that's not practical, then whisper the words. If that's awkward too, then do the best you can.

Seven-by-Seven works. (Many of Dr. Goljan's patients have gotten positive results in a matter of days.) You shouldn't repeat the four answers *fewer* than seven times in a row, seven times a day; doing it *more* than that may make it more effective.

Once you stop clenching and grinding your teeth, you can stop doing the Seven-by-Seven system. But you have to realize that the bad pattern will always be in your subconscious. If given the opportunity—the setup of stressful conditions—that old pattern may raise its ugly head. It is for that reason, Dr. Goljan wisely suggests, you do a day or two of the Seven-by-Seven every two weeks or maybe once a month to reinforce the new programming.

If Dr. Goljan's Seven-by-Seven system works for you, you can apply it to *everything* in your life that's a problem.

P.S. We have a friend who grinds his teeth at night. So, before he goes to bed, he fills his mouth with coffee beans and sets his clock for eight. But seriously . . .

At bedtime, chew two chewable calcium tablets. Make sure the label specifies "chewable."

GUM PROBLEMS

Thanks to TV commercials, "gingivitis" has become a common word for an even more common condition. If you have gingivitis—red, swollen, bleeding gums—there are treatments that can help. Herbs, tinctures, and vitamins mentioned below are available at most health food stores.

In order to get positive results, you must keep at it daily—morning, noon (if possible), and night—

• Myrrh, as a tincture or in powder form, can be used effectively to heal gums. Add a teaspoon of myrrh tincture to two tablespoons of water. Hold it in your mouth for three minutes, then spit it out. Or, wet your toothbrush and pour a little powdered myrrh on it, then gently but firmly massage the gums. Do it two to three times a day, starting first thing in the morning and last thing at night.

• There are a combination of garlic and parsley extract capsules. Take two every four hours for at least three days.

• Add a teaspoon of tincture of calendula to two tablespoons of water. Hold it in your mouth for three minutes, then spit it out. Do it two to three times a day, starting first thing in the morning and last thing at night.

• Use bee propolis as a toothpaste, and/or dissolve five drops of propolis in a half-glass of water and ration out this milky drink throughout the day.

• In addition to any of the above, take vitamin C (500 mgs) twice a day.

Tartar Prevention: This is for those of you who have problems even though you take great care of your teeth and gums—always brushing after meals, flossing, and gum-massaging, in addition to staying away from sugary foods and eating raw, firm, and fibrous vegetables daily.

To help stop the formation of problem-causing tartar, take two papaya pills after every meal. Keep one pill on each side of your mouth and just let it dissolve. It can kill bacteria, rid you of dead gum tissue, and help digestion, too.

FOR DENTURE WEARERS

Denture-Sore Gums: Massage sore gums with tincture of myrrh (available at health food stores), or put a half-teaspoon of the myrrh tincture in a cup of warm water and use it as a mouthwash.

Denture Cleanser: Keep your dentures clean by soaking them overnight in a cup of white vinegar.

Dentures and Gas: If you have more gas than usual and you can't figure out why, check the fit of your dentures. Ill-fitting dentures can cause you to swallow lots of air, thus the additional gas.

Keep Dentures Fitting Better Longer: As the years pass after you've gotten dentures, your jawbone shrinks. That shrinking process can throw off the proper fit of your dentures. To slow down and minimize the jawbone shrinkage, eat foods rich in vitamin D—bone meal, tuna, sardines, salmon, herring, cod, and milk and milk products. Also eat foods high in calcium—steamed leafy green vegetables (collard, dandelion, mustard), sesame seeds, sardines, cheddar cheese, Swiss cheese, and seaweed. You can also supplement your diet with vitamin D and calcium pills. Ask your health professional for the dosage that's appropriate for you.

A sad reminder: The absorption of calcium is blocked by eating chocolate.

BAD BREATH

If you're troubled by occasional bad breath and you know it's not a symptom of indigestion, gum disease, or anything other than occasional bad breath, these suggestions may help—

• Dip two sprigs of parsley in white vinegar and chew it, chew it, chew it.

• Mix three drops of peppermint oil in a glass of warm water. Take a mouthful, swish it around your mouth, and spit it out;

take another mouthful and gargle with it, then spit it out. Keep doing that until you finish the glassful.

• Chew a few fennel seeds, dill seeds, or hazelnuts.

• Every time you brush your teeth, brush the bacteria, minute food particles, and toxins off your tongue, too. Use your toothbrush or scrape your tongue with a teaspoon or commercial tongue-scraper sold in health food stores. A dozen brushes or scrapes from back to front ought to do it.

DRY MOUTH

Almost half of all Americans over age fifty-five have a dry mouth. Daily use of prescription drugs can cause the problem. What to do?

• If possible, take a sip of water every few minutes.

• Suck on sugar-free hard candies.

• Chew your tongue. Within half a minute, you should be able to manufacture enough saliva to relieve the dryness.

This is one of those conditions where we urge you to try these remedies with your doctor's supervision. Promise. C'mon, promise. I'll be your best friend. Actually, you should be your own best friend and take good care of yourself. That means, professional medical overseeing when it comes to ulcers.

The most prevalent misconception about ulcers is that milk is soothing; spicy foods can kill you. Wrong! There *is* controversy about the benefits of milk. Let me put it this way . . . There are many more healing foods than milk—spicy foods, for instance. You read that right.

• Cayenne (red) pepper is thought to be one of the most helpful spices when it comes to ulcer-healing and, in the process, it dulls the pains. It's strong and may take getting used to. Start with one-eighth teaspoon of cayenne pepper in a glass of water twice a day. Gradually work your way up to a quarter-teaspoon.

If you just can't take it, capsules are available at health food stores. Take three a day right after eating.

• A Chinese stomach ulcer remedy calls for diet changes: Eliminate fried foods, flour products (that means "no bread"), alcoholic beverages, and smoking.

In addition to the dietary no-nos, have one teaspoon of olive oil before each meal, and end your day with a tablespoon of powdered alfalfa in a glass of water.

• A cup of catnip tea before each meal has worked wonders for many with stomach ulcers. Prepare the tea by steeping a teaspoon of catnip (available at health food stores) in a cup of just-boiled water. After five minutes, strain and drink.

Cats are crazy about this herb and will go to great lengths to get at it. If you have a cat and you plan to use this remedy, keep the catnip in a tightly sealed sturdy container. No fooling.

• First thing in the morning, paint the soles of your feet with apple cider vinegar. Let them dry naturally before putting on socks or hose. Put on another layer of vinegar right before dinner. Just do it. Humor us and see if it works, then let us know.

• The classic ulcer folk remedy is raw cabbage. The contemporary version of this remedy is raw cabbage *juice.* To prepare the juice, you will need a juice extractor. It can be expensive, but it's a wise investment considering the healthful drinks you can make with it.

For ulcers, juice and drink a half-cup of fresh cabbage juice before each meal and a half-cup at bedtime. If you hate the taste, add some fresh carrot juice. Since it's not advisable to juice the cabbage in advance—which means it may not be practical for you to have it before each meal when you're out of the house and not near a juicer—do the best you can and have it as often as possible.

Within a few weeks, don't be surprised if your doctor tells you there's no trace of an ulcer.

• During the last few years, we've received the same remedies from several people who used to have ulcers. The key words here are, "used to have ulcers." Their remedy consisted of aloe vera juice (available at health food stores), one tablespoon after each meal.

• My friend's mother was diagnosed as having an ulcer. She decided to make barley and barley water a major part of her daily diet. The results were terrific. In fact, her doctor was so impressed with the fast healing, he now recommends barley to other ulcer patients.

Boil two ounces of barley in six cups of water. When there's about half of the water left—three cups—take it off the fire. Strain and let the liquid cool. Add buckwheat honey to taste. Buckwheat honey is wonderful for ulcer sufferers. It can help neutralize stomach acid and soothe delicate membranes of the digestive tract. With or without honey, have at least three cups of barley water a day.

You can eat the barley as a side dish or in soup or stew, but drinking the barley water is most important.

• Propolis is a sticky substance collected by bees from the buds of certain trees. Bees use it to help hold their hive together. People can use propolis to help heal ulcers. You can get propolis extract, tablets, or capsules at most health food stores. Take 500 mgs three times a day until the condition clears up completely.

𝒮 **Affirmation:** Repeat this affirmation three times in a row. *I let go of my anxiety and my anger; I replace it with love and harmony.*
Each time you say the affirmation, start with your fists clenched and up against your chest. When you say "I let go . . . ," thrust your arms and fingers out into the air in front of you. When you say, "I replace it with . . . ," bring your arms back in, hugging yourself. Go through this process first thing in the morning, whenever you walk into a room and no one else is there (doesn't that happen each time you go to the bathroom?), and last thing at night.

URINARY AND
KIDNEY PROBLEMS

The urinary tract consists of all organs and ducts involved in the release and elimination of urine.

As part of the urinary tract, the average adult bladder holds twenty-four ounces of urine. When the walls of the bladder are stretched, nerve impulses trigger the urge to urinate. That usually happens when the bladder has ten to sixteen ounces of urine.

The two kidneys, shaped like kidney beans and located in the back of the abdomen, on each side of the spine, are the principal organs of the urinary system. The kidneys filter the blood—all of it—once an hour.

The urinary system is an extraordinarily sophisticated one and, as with all complex machinery, things can go wrong. Because this is a serious subject, and an accurate diagnosis is all-important, consult a health professional as soon as you suspect a urinary problem. If you plan to use any of these home remedies, check with that health professional first.

URINARY PROBLEMS

Urinary Tract Infection: Drink a cup of cranberry juice daily . . . if your doctor hasn't already suggested it.

Frequent Urination: If you have the urge to go every two minutes, long before your bladder could have accumulated the appropriate ounces of urine, try this string bean remedy.

Clean a half-pound of string beans, put them in a pot, and cover them with water, then add another cup of water. Cover the pot and cook the string beans for ten minutes. Once a day, on an empty stomach, eat the string beans and the water they were cooked in.

A Chinese remedy for stopping the frequent urge to urinate is to eat three fresh, uncooked chestnuts before breakfast and three after dinner. (Use a nutcracker to help you open and peel them.) Take your time and chew them thoroughly.

Painful Urination: Aloe vera juice can help heal an inflamed bladder that may cause painful urination. Take a jigger of aloe vera first thing in the morning and right after your evening meal.

𝒮 **Affirmation and Visualization:** Be seated in a comfortable chair. After you say this affirmation just once, take seven slow, deep breaths. As you take each one, visualize the air you're inhaling as blue-white healing energy. Feel it flowing through your body, repairing whatever needs to be repaired. Do this affirming/visualizing process first thing in the morning— maybe even before you get out of bed—and do it once at coffee-break time in the afternoon, and again before you go to sleep.

I release my anger and I relax. With each breath I take, healing energy enters my body, flows through me, and I am better and better.

KIDNEY PROBLEMS

Kidney and Bladder Infection: Flaxseed (available at health food stores) can help fight an infection. Prepare tea by steeping one tablespoon of flaxseed in one pint of just-boiled water. After seven minutes, strain out the flaxseed if you're watching your weight (flaxseed can increase one's appetite). If that's not a concern, or if you're at all constipated, then eat the flaxseed. Most important for the kidney and bladder infection is that you drink the two cups of flaxseed tea daily.

Kidney Detoxifier: Parsnip is a great detoxifier. It can help clean out your kidneys, and may even promote the passing of stones.

One serving of parsnip is not going to do the trick. We're

talking about eating parsnip at least twice a day for at least a week. Steam it, grill it, or bake it, and eat it!

Kidney Stone Dissolvers: Constant sips of liquid are essential for flushing the kidneys and helping dissolve stones. Consult with your doctor to decide which drink(s) are best for you—

Fresh parsley juice has been used with success to dissolve kidney stones. To sweeten the strong green taste of the parsley, add fresh carrot juice.

For a little variety, you may want to drink cranberry juice. Not only does it help with most urinary problems, but it also can help dissolve kidney stones.

Watermelon seed tea (available at health food stores) is a wonderful diuretic and kidney cleanser.

These are herb teas that have been known to dissolve kidney stones—sometimes within hours. Several cups must be consumed to get results. This is where a health professional can guide you to the right herb and dosage. These teas are

- Camomile
- Buchu
- Cornsilk—fresh or dried
- Uva Ursi—also called bearberry

Passing the Kidney Stones: When you suspect that you might pass a stone or gravel, urinate through unbleached muslin or a linen handkerchief—or into a chamber pot—so you can catch it. It's important to turn the stone over to your doctor. Analysis of it can help you prevent a recurrence of the problem. For instance, the stones may be oxalatic, which means you should stay away from spinach, rhubarb, almonds, and cashews. The stones may show an excess of dietary calcium, or too much vitamin D, or they can be uric acid stones caused by gout medicine.

Kidney Stone Prevention: Eating two tablespoons of rice bran can help prevent kidney stones. Sprinkle it on salads, in soups, and stews. You can also stir it in juice or shakes.

Gem Therapy: Bloodstone is recommended. Hold it and rub it, wear it, carry it with you, or tape it to your body—the area on your back that's closest to your kidneys.

S **Affirmation:** Repeat this fifteen times a day, starting first thing in the morning, every time you urinate, and last thing at night—

As my fears melt away, I am empowered by the unlimited good that's out there for me.

VAGINITIS

The three most common types of vaginitis are yeast, tricho-monal, and bacterial infections. Chances are you will need pro-fessional help to determine the kind of infection you have and the severity of it. If you are put on antibiotics, be sure to take acidophilus, available at health food stores (the capsules should have one to two billion viable acidophilus cells; read the label carefully). The antibiotics have no discretion; they destroy the good as well as the bad bacteria. Therefore you must take acidophilus to replace the beneficial bacteria.

Take the acidophilus right after you've eaten and at least two hours before or two hours after you take an antibiotic. That way you won't make the antibiotic crazy going after the benefi-cial bacteria in the acidophilus.

Once the antibiotic does its job and rids you of the infection, we'd like to help you prevent it from recurring. Here are some suggestions—

• Wear loose-fitting cotton panties. Cut the crotch out of your panty hose. Wear skirts; stay away from tight-fitting slacks or jeans.

• Launder with unscented detergent. Do not use bleach or fabric softener. They can irritate sensitive skin.

• Iron those cotton panties to make sure all bacteria are destroyed.

• Sleep without panties.

• When you go to the bathroom, *always* wipe from front to back.

- Do not wash the vagina with soap. The natural pH balance can be unbalanced by soap, which is usually alkaline, leaving you more susceptible to infection.

- Garlic is a natural antibiotic. Add garlic to your diet—raw garlic is, by far, best.

- If a yeast infection is your problem, eliminate processed sugar from your diet immediately. There are good books available detailing a yeast-free diet.

At the Onset of Vaginitis or for Mild Cases: This remedy was given to us by a gynecologist in Chicago. He said that douching twice a day with pau d'arco can greatly ease the symptoms or rid you completely of the infection. The herb is also called le pacho and taheebo and is available at health food stores and herb shops.

Vaginal Itching: Garlic will stop the itching in most cases. To prepare garlic water, dice six cloves of garlic and put them in a quart of just-boiled water. Cover it and let it steep for twenty minutes. Strain and wash the genital area with liquid and douche with it.

Or, break open two or three acidophilus capsules (available at health food stores) and mix with enough vegetable oil to form a runny paste. Gently smear it on the sore, itchy area. It should stop the itching quickly and start healing the irritated skin.

𝒮 **Affirmation:** Repeat this affirmation ten times a day, first thing in the morning, each time you comb or brush your hair, and last thing at night—

I accept myself as a healthy and happy woman, blessed with normal and natural bodily functions.

❧ VARICOSE VEINS ❧

One of every two women past the age of forty has varicose veins. As for men in the same age bracket, one out of every four has the problem.

If you are one of the millions with varicose veins, we have some helpful suggestions. If you don't have them yet, I'm surprised you're reading this chapter. But, good for you. You may want to take these preventive measures—

•   Do not cross your legs when you sit. Women: For a graceful, feminine look, sit with your knees together and your legs slanted to the side.

•   Do not wear socks, hose, or garters that will constrict the blood flow at any point on your legs.

•   Take at least 200 mgs of vitamin C daily. It will help keep your veins in shape.

•   Exercise daily—walking is great; so is bicycling or swimming.

•   Elevate your legs for a half hour a day, making sure your feet are about four inches higher than your heart. Any time you can sit with your legs elevated, do so.

VARICOSE VEINS REMEDIES:

For those who already suffer from this condition, exercise and elevation of the legs are extremely important in the healing process. The following remedies are also helpful—

•   Savoy cabbage leaves can be very healing, particularly in severe cases of varicose veins. Take a few leaves, cut away the outer part, and iron the spine in the center . . . yes, with a regular iron. Since there's no setting for "vegetables," set it for "wool." The leaves should then be soft and flat. Put them on the veins and bind them in place with an Ace bandage. Or, if you have support stockings that are large enough to wear over the cabbage leaves, that would be good. Wear them all day and/or overnight. Do it daily and watch for an improvement along with relief.

• Vitamin E can help eliminate varicose veins. Please remember that even with vitamins, more is not always better. Check with your health professional for dosage that's appropriate for you.

• Drink two cups of oatstraw tea daily. Prepare the tea by steeping a teaspoon of oatstraw (available at health food stores) into a cup of just-boiled water. Ten minutes later, strain and drink.

Once a week, take an oatstraw bath. Steep one third of a cup of oatstraw in a quart of just-boiled water, strain, and pour the liquid into your warm bath water. Relax and enjoy it for at least twenty minutes.

• For varicose ulcers, prepare a poultice using cod liver oil and an equal amount of raw honey. Bind it in place overnight, every night, until the condition clears up.

 Affirmation: Repeat this affirmation fifteen times a day, starting first thing in the morning, every time you remind yourself to elevate your legs, and last thing at night—

Healing energy is flowing freely through my veins as I move through life with ease.

For as many warts as there are in this world, that's how many remedies there seem to be for their removal. Remedies range from sensible to something out of the "Twilight Zone."

No other ailment (it *is* a virus, you know) is as rich in folklore as warts. Through the years, we've accumulated quite a collection (of folklore, that is). Most recently we were told: Rub the wart with a stolen egg, then wrap the egg in brown paper, and leave it at a crossroads. When someone picks up the package and breaks the egg, you will get rid of the wart and that person will get it.

One of our favorites is an old Irish remedy: Collect a little mound of dirt under your right foot and kick it toward a passing hearse as you chant: "Oh corpse of clay, as you decay, come and carry my wart away."

The odd part about some of these outrageous remedies is that they actually work. It's a perfect example of the power of suggestion.

We have some powerful suggestions that mostly fall in the "sensible" category. When using any of them, be consistent and be patient. For common warts—

• Dab apple cider vinegar on the wart, and before it dries, put on baking soda, too. Dust off the soda after 15 minutes. Do this a half-dozen times a day, every day, until the wart disappears.

• Put a piece of raw eggplant on the wart and keep it in place overnight with an Ace bandage. If you can walk around with the eggplant on the wart during the day, do so. If not, put on a fresh piece of raw eggplant every night until the wart is gone.

• Smother the wart with oil—wheat germ oil, castor oil, vitamin E oil, vitamin A, or oil of cinnamon.

At the start of your day, after your morning shower, drench a cotton ball with the oil of your choice, apply it to the wart, and keep it in place with a Band-Aid. Do the same thing at bedtime. Within a month of oiling the wart twice a day, it should be history.

• This is a little "Twilight Zone–ish," but it was given to us by a level-headed lady who was as skeptical as you probably will be, until it worked for her:

Cut an apple into as many pieces as there are warts. Assign each slice to a wart and rub that slice on its wart. After doing that, put the apple back together and bury it. When the apple rots, the warts will be gone.

• This remedy, taken with any of the above remedies, is thought to speed up the wart-drying process.

Prepare fresh or frozen asparagus and purée it in a blender. Eat one-fourth cup of the purée twice a day—before breakfast and before dinner.

Warts Under and Around Fingernails: Take medical adhesive tape and wrap it around the warted finger four times. Make sure it's airless and secure, but not so tight as to stop the circulation. After a week, before bedtime, take off the tape and sleep without it. Next morning re-dress the finger again and leave it on for another week. Keep up this pattern and by the end of the third or fourth week the wart should weaken, wither, and waste away.

Warts on Hands: We love it when people send us success stories. Lisa Jade had a wart on the palm of her hand. Her dermatologist tried liquid nitrogen on it. At first it was a little better, but then the pain and size increased. Lisa went to another doctor who gave her a prescription that didn't help much either. Then, after seeing us on TV, she ran to the mall, bought our book, *More Chicken Soup,* and tried our remedy—

Boil a couple of eggs and save the water. As soon as the water cools, soak your warted hand in that water for ten minutes. Do it daily until the wart disappears.

Lisa said that all it took was *one* soaking for the pain and the wart to vanish, leaving no trace of it whatsoever.

Genital Warts: There's good news and there's bad news. The good news is that you are not alone; this is a common problem. The bad news is that it's a common problem because genital warts are quite contagious. So, refrain (if we have to tell you from what, then you're already refraining) until the warts disappear. Meanwhile—

Squeeze out a vitamin E and/or vitamin A capsule and apply. Since warmth and moisture encourage the growth of warts, do not put a Band-Aid on it; just keep reapplying the oil as often as possible each day until you abort the wart.

Or, gently rub the wart with a piece of fresh, ripe pineapple. Do it at least twice a day—the more often, the better.

Plantar Warts: Get a basin big enough for your foot. Every night, fill the basin with one gallon of warm water and a half cup of Arm & Hammer Super Washing Soda and soak your foot for fifteen minutes. Then rub dry the sole of your foot with a rough washcloth. At some point, little black spots will appear. They're the roots of the warts and they will come out and off, never to return. The entire process takes about two weeks.

Or try this remedy: At bedtime each night, take one or two vitamin A or garlic capsules, puncture them, and squeeze out the oil on the plantar warts. Massage the oil on the whole area for a few minutes—do a thorough job. Then, after you've let it set for a few more minutes, put a clean, white sock on your foot and sleep that way. This, as with most wart remedies, takes about two weeks for results.

Finally, you might soak your foot in a basin of hot water for five minutes every night. Then soak a cotton ball with Listerine, apply it directly on the plantar warts, and tape it in place. (Listerine? Who discovered this? Maybe it was someone who was used to putting his foot in his mouth.) After one or two weeks, the warts should be gone, leaving your foot kissing sweet.

Visualization: Upon rising and at bedtime, sit up in bed (if you prefer, sit on a hard-back chair), and close your eyes for a two- to three-minute visualization.

Start by breathing out all the air in your lungs, then slowly breathing in. As you exhale, visualize a huge theater marquee with bright lights flashing the number "3" three times. Take another slow, deep breath, and as you exhale, visualize the number "2" flashing three times. Take one more deep breath, slowly, and when you exhale, see the number "1" flashing three times.

Now that you're relaxed and ready, visualize your refrigerator. Open the door and on the top shelf see a colorful artist's palette. Pick up the palette, and the magical gold paintbrush that's alongside of it. Don't forget to close the refrigerator door. Now visualize the wart and the area that surrounds it. As you hold the palette in one hand and the brush in your other hand, the brush will magically dip into the color on the palette that matches your skin tone perfectly. Take the brush and paint over the wart—keep re-dipping the brush and continue painting the wart until the wart completely disappears.

Slowly count from one to three. Open your eyes, stretch, and feel refreshed.

𝒮 **Affirmation:** Cover the wart with something—a tissue, your sleeve, your hand—then repeat this affirmation at least twelve times a day, first thing in the morning, last thing at night, and right before you drink any beverage—

I have positive feelings. Everything in my life is clear and wonderful.

Reducing Inducement: Find something portable weighing ten, fifteen, maybe twenty pounds. Keep it with you for a full day. Don't make a move without it. See what it's like carrying around the extra weight. That just may be the motivation you need to lose those excess pounds.

The following tips, tricks, and tactics can help you eat less and feel satisfied sooner—

• Drink tomato juice about fifteen minutes before you eat. The acid in the juice can give you a full feeling, making it possible to eat smaller portions than usual without feeling deprived.

• Put one tablespoon of apple cider vinegar and two tablespoons of honey in a glass of unsweetened grapefruit juice. Mix thoroughly and drink it a half hour before each meal. In addition to reducing your appetite, this drink is said to help regulate your thyroid and melt fat away, too.

• Right before you start to eat, tighten your belt a notch—not enough to make your eyes bulge, but just enough to make you feel full sooner than usual.

• Turn off the rock-and-roll music while at the table. It makes you eat faster and more.

• Drink a glass of water before each meal. It helps flush your system and give you a full feeling. It can also cut down on a craving, which may unknowingly have been for water to begin with. If just the glass of water doesn't work for you, you may want to try eating half of a ripe (brown speckled) banana before you drink the water. That can be very filling.

• This New Age/Age-Old yoga tip can be a real conversation starter at a dinner table. When you eat, plug up your left nostril so that you breathe through your right nostril only. It is said that this process speeds up metabolism and allows you to quickly and efficiently derive all the energy from the food you eat. And so, you don't have to eat as much as usual to be satisfied.

THE BENEFITS OF EXERCISE

You need it! We *all* need it! Yes, exercise burns calories. A brisk forty-five-minute walk burns 300 calories. Do that every day and you can lose eighteen pounds in a year.

Some fitness experts believe that when you exercise right before you eat, you rev up your metabolism and it stays *revved* for a while, helping you to metabolize your food faster and more effectively. Exercise also helps cleanse your system by stimulating the elimination of wastes.

In addition to your regular workouts or walkouts, each time there's a commercial break on television, stand up, stretch, and exercise, even if it's just dancing to music in the commercials. This serves several purposes: It gets the circulation going; burns some calories; and, most important, it keeps you out of the kitchen!

And did you know that finger-drumming, toe-tapping, seat-squirming, and other forms of fidgeting can burn off big-time calories? In a twenty-four-hour period, fidgeters who were tested used up as many as 800 calories, compared to non-fidgeters who used up only 100 calories for "spontaneous physical activity," during the same period of time.

Trigger Foods: There are trigger foods—just one bite *triggers* an out-of-control binge. They generally fall into the category of sugary, fatty, high-cholesterol, or salty foods. After all, who binges on broccoli?

Do you have one or more trigger foods? Think about it. Identify the foods. Realize the consequences of compulsive eating that trigger foods cause. Eliminate the trigger foods from your life and you eliminate temptation, demoralization, and other negative and unhealthy repercussions.

"Sweet Tooth" Substitutes:

A very overweight person went to the doctor. After a thorough examination, the doctor told the patient, "You need a bypass." "A bypass?" "Yes. Bypass the refrigerator, bypass the bakery, bypass desserts . . ."

• Dissolve a teaspoon of baking soda in a glass of warm water and rinse your mouth with it. Within a few minutes, probably by the time you're down to the last mouthful of the mixture, your taste buds will be appeased and the something-sweet urge will be submerged.

• Boil an artichoke for ten to fifteen minutes and eat it— without butter. It's plenty good that way. And since it has a fructose-derived substance called inulin (not insulin), it fills the desire for something sweet.

• Stir a heaping teaspoon or two of brewer's yeast (available at health food stores) in a glass of unsweetened grapefruit juice. Drink this mixture before each meal. It may help you eat less during the meal and it should help you conquer your sweet tooth completely within a few days.

Helpful Herbs: These herbs (available at health food stores) can help curb your appetite, quell your cravings, and flush out the fat cells. Stick with one herb and be sure to pay attention to your reaction to it. Do you seem to be less hungry? Do you have more control over your desire to snack? After a few days, change to another herb and note your responses to it. Keep doing this until you've tried all the herbs and know which does what for you.

Prepare herbal tea by steeping a teaspoon of the herb in a cup of just-boiled water. After seven minutes, strain and sip slowly.

- • Hawthorn berry tea—two cups daily
- • Psyllium seed husks tea—one to two cups daily (it's a good colon cleanser, so stay close to home)
- • Chaparral tea—three cups daily, one after each meal
- • Lady's mantle tea—two to three cups daily
- • Chicory root tea—one cup daily before breakfast
- • Chickweed tea—three cups daily, one before each meal

Nature's Best Diet Food: Research reports say that bee pollen can correct body metabolism imbalances, stimulate the metabolic processes, and speed up the burning of calories. It's said to eliminate cravings and act as an appetite suppressant. The lecithin in bee pollen is known to dissolve and flush fat from the body. Bee pollen promises a lot and, from our research, we have reason to believe it delivers. In fact, both of us recently started taking bee pollen every day. If you're interested in trying it, begin with just a few granules for the first couple of days, to make sure you don't have an allergy to it. If there's no allergic reaction, take a quarter-teaspoon for a few days. Gradually work your way up to a teaspoon a day. Some people get results on only a teaspoon a day; others need to work their way up to a tablespoon a day.

Nature's Thyroid Booster: Add a tablespoon of seaweed to soup, stew, or salad every day. Kelp is the most popular seaweed and is available at health food stores. According to Dr. J. W. Turentine, a scientist with the U.S. Department of Agriculture, "Of the fourteen elements essential to the proper metabolic functions of the human body, thirteen are known to be in kelp." One of the thirteen elements is organic iodine, which rouses the thyroid gland into action, stimulating the body's metabolism and, ultimately, turns fatty foods into energy.

Aromatherapy: According to Alan R. Hirsch, M.D., neurologist, psychiatrist, and director of the Smell and Taste Treatment and Research Foundation, "The stronger the flavor of the food, the stronger its power to satisfy and reduce hunger. The odor of a hearty Greek salad topped with a spicy vinaigrette dressing, a strong cheese, and some anchovies will do wonders to decrease appetite in a hurry."

Dr. Hirsch's findings are based on extensive research. He advises dieters, "Sniff each bite of food quickly five times before eating. Fast sniffs signal food messages to the brain that decrease hunger and work to satisfy appetite without calories. Opt for hot foods. The heat and steam from the food send flavor molecules up the back of the throat and into the brain satiety center faster."

Dr. Hirsch says, "Don't snack between meals. Sniff! Keep a chocolate bar in your desk at work. When the urge for chocolate takes hold, sniff the candy. The smell of food can trick your body into thinking you've already eaten."

One more tip from Dr. Hirsch: "When drinking beverages, blow bubbles in the drink with a straw before sipping. By doing so, the odors of the liquid emanate into the nasal passages to satisfy hunger."

Gem Therapy: If food addiction is your problem, you might want to consider amethyst, the stone for addictive behavior, substance abuse, and for any dependencies.

If you use food as an escape or avoidance technique, carnelian may be the stone for you. It is said to help you focus on the present. When you're "here now," chances are you won't want to use food as a diversion. So, wear or carry amethyst and/or carnelian to help you control a weight problem.

Visualization and Affirmation: This is not a typical visualization process. It's more of an arts and crafts assignment.

Find a photo of yourself—if possible, one of you smiling. Then go through magazines and find a figure you would like to have and that's in proportion to the photo of you. Put the picture of your head on that body, and place it where you will see it often: on the refrigerator, on your desk, alongside your television set.

When you walk away from the picture, repeat this affirmation seven times, while visualizing the picture you just saw.

I am someone special. I love me and I'm creating the life I want.

REFERRALS

For information about smell and taste disorders, and aromatherapy research, write or call:

Dr. Alan R. Hirsch
Smell & Taste Research Foundation Ltd.
Water Tower Place Suite 990W
845 No. Michigan Avenue

Chicago, IL 60611
312/938-1047

For a referral to a local chapter of a nonprofit fellowship of
men and women who share their experience, strength, and
hope with each other that they may solve their common
problem and help others to recover from compulsive overeating, write to or call:

Overeaters Anonymous
World Service Office
P.O. Box 44020
Rio Rancho, NM 87174-4020
505/891-2664
Fax: 505/891-4320

A Healthy Auric Field: Barbara Brennan, faith healer, physicist, and psychotherapist, describes our auric field as the field of bioenergy that runs through and around the body. The more powerfully charged, balanced, and clear it is, the stronger your immune system is and the less susceptible you are to illness. According to Barbara—

• The sun charges the auric field. Get sun for ten to twenty minutes a day.

• Don't work under fluorescent lights. They have a negative impact on the auric field.

• Eliminate negative thoughts. They create an imbalance in the auric field. To erase negative thoughts, figure out what's causing them and take action to eliminate the problem. Don't just put the blame for your negative thoughts on others and attempt to live with the problem.

Color It Healing: Laurie Zagon, internationally known artist and color authority, says that the universal healing color is turquoise—a combination of blue and green. It is healing for the person who wears turquoise and for people who see it being worn.

Jokes and Laughter: Share laughter and you can make new friends or improve and deepen the level of communication with old friends, family members, and business associates.

Make a real effort to lighten up. Be playful. Have fun. It can make a major difference in your sense of well-being and in your relationship with everyone in your life.

In this day and age, there are tons of things to tickle your funny bone. There are books, television shows, video cassettes, audio cassettes, comedy clubs across the country, and the funniest of all, real life. Seek and ye shall find the humor surrounding you.

Are you game? Good. Tell a joke to the next person you see or speak to. If you're one of those people who says, "I can't tell a joke," tell it anyway. It'd probably be funnier than told by someone with a slick delivery. So that you don't have the I-don't-know-any-joke excuse, here are a few to choose from. (Who knows, this may start you on a whole new career, but for the time being, hold onto your day job.)

JOKE #1: An elderly man goes to the doctor and complains, "Every time I want to make love to my wife, nothing happens. Doctor, you've got to help me!" The doctor examines the man and finds that everything is in good working order. After asking his patient some questions, the doctor discovers the problem. "Mr. Newman, you sit around the house all day and that makes you tired. What you need is exercise. Daily exercise will stimulate your system, wake up your organs, and get those old juices flowing again." Mr. Newman is willing to try it. The doctor tells him to walk ten miles a day. As Mr. Newman is leaving the office, the doctor tells him, "Remember, ten miles a day and call me in a week with a progress report." A week later, when Mr. Newman calls, the doctor asks, "Did you walk ten miles a day like I said?" His patient answers, "Yes. I said I would and I did." The doctor's next question is, "And did you make love to your wife?" Mr. Newman says, "How can I? I'm seventy miles from home!"

JOKE #2: Do you know why the Siamese twins moved to London? *(Pause)* So that the other one could drive. (If you don't get a laugh, say—"Think about it.")

JOKE #3: (Everyone loves a lawyer joke . . . even lawyers.) A lawyer died and went to heaven. As soon as St. Peter saw him, he swung open the Pearly Gates and the celebration began. There was a parade, marching bands, banners waving, food, and drink. The lawyer said to St. Peter, "Excuse me, but I think there's some kind of mistake. I was just an ordinary lawyer. I didn't do anything special for humankind. I made no major contribution." St. Peter said, "Oh, but it's not every day we get someone who's a hundred and twenty-seven years old." The lawyer corrected St. Peter, "I was only sixty-four when I died." "Not according to your billable hours," answered St. Peter.

Take advantage of one of the greatest gifts of being human. Laugh!

If you're among the fifteen percent of the American population with no sense of humor, you might consider joining the National Association for the Humor Impaired, founded by Dr. Stuart Robertshaw, psychology professor at the University of Wisconsin-La Crosse. More information in the Referral.

Healing Music: Spirited music can improve blood circulation and boost muscular strength and endurance. Your favorite music can make the most arduous task seem almost pleasant. Soothing music can keep blood pressure down, help you sleep, and get you out of a funk.

According to *The Compass in Your Nose and Other Astonishing Facts About Humans* (Jeremy P. Tarcher, Inc., 1989), musical scores that approximate the rhythm of the resting heart (seventy beats per minute) can actually slow a heart that is beating too fast. The music found most effective in slowing an anxious heart includes:

- Venus, the Bringer of Peace (The Planets), by Holst

- Mother Goose Suite, first movement, by Ravel

- The Brandenburg Concertos, No. 4, Second Movement, by Bach

- Orchestral Suite, No. 2 (Saraband), by Bach

The Pet Set: Research suggests that people who have pets are generally happier and healthier than those without animal companions.

Studies at the University of California-Davis show that elderly people with pets feel more secure, have a more positive outlook and attitude, and they exercise more than their petless peers.

And what better way to meet new people than by walking a dog . . . no matter how old you are?

Reach Out and Touch Someone: We need to be touched. It's a human requirement as basic as food and air. It's been proven with infants who are deprived of touch and sadly wither away. Now, researchers are discovering that adults have the same need for touch and can benefit from it as much as infants.

Of course you've got to use discretion and touch people in an appropriate and acceptable way. A pat on the back for someone you work with; a pinch on the cheek when someone says something adorable; a good old-fashioned hug when you're very proud of a friend or family member. If you're not thought of as a touchy-feely person, a hug out of the blue from you may frighten the intended recipient. If that's the case, you should consider some kind of friendly warning like, "I feel a hug coming on."

If you are sincere and congruent about touching someone, that touch will be appreciated by that lucky person. Actually, it will make you both feel better.

♫ **Affirmation:** Repeat this affirmation seven times, starting first thing in the morning, every time you get a negative feeling, and last thing at night.

I am happy, healthy, and safe. My life is filled with sunshine, laughter, and love.

REFERRAL

For a "Quick Score Test for Humor Impairment," and membership in the National Association for the Humor Impaired, write about one of the funniest things that ever happened to you (keep it brief) and send it to:

Professor Stuart Robertshaw
National Association for the Humor Impaired
400 South 15th Street Suite 201
La Crosse, WI 54601

Resources

Here is a list of companies who offer catalogs for a wide variety of helpful products and information.

Herbal Products and More

Blessed Herbs
109 Barre Plains Road
Oakham, MA 01068

Free catalog
800/489-4372

Great American Natural Products
4121 16th Street North
St. Petersburg, FL 33703

Free catalog
800/323-4372

Old Amish Herbal Remedies
4141 Irish Street North
St. Petersburg, FL 33703

Free catalog
813/521-4372

Penn Herb Co. Ltd.
603 North 2nd Street
Philadelphia, PA 19123

Free catalog
800/523-9971

Haussmann's Pharmacy
534–536 West Girard Avenue
Philadelphia, PA 19123

Free catalog
800/235-5522
215/627-2143

Nature's Apothecary
997 Dixon Road
Boulder, CO 80303

Free catalog
800/999-7422
303/440-7422

New Chapter, Inc. Free catalog
P.O. Box 1947 800/543-7279
99 Main Street 802/257-0018
Brattleboro, VT 05301

Mountain Rose Herbs Free catalog
P.O. Box 2000 800/879-3337
Redway, CA 95560 707/923-7867

Health Center for Better Living Free catalog
6189 Taylor Road 800/544-4225
Naples, FL 33942

Dial Herbs Free catalog
P.O. Box 39 800/288-4618
Fairview, UT 84629 801/427-9476

Indiana Botanic Gardens Free catalog
P.O. Box 5 800/644-8327
Hammond, IN 46325 219/947-4040

Aphrodisia Send SASE for
282 Bleecker Street Herb List
New York, NY 10014 212/989-6440

Bee Products and More

CC Pollen Co. Free catalog
Suite 209 800/950-0096
3627 East Indian School Road
Phoenix, AZ 85018-5126

Montana Naturals International Inc. Free catalog
19994 Highway 93 800/872-7218
Arlee, MT 59821

Ginseng Products and More

Hsu's Ginseng Enterprises, Inc. Free catalog
T 6819 County Highway West 800/388-3818
P.O. Box 509 715/675-2325
Wausau, WI 54402-0509

Products for Allergy Relief, Antioxidants, and More

NutriCology, Inc. (Allergy Research Group)   Free catalog
400 Preda Street   800/545-9960
San Leandro, CA 94577

Health-Related Products

Home Health Products, Inc.   Free catalog
P.O. Box 8425   800/284-9123
Virginia Beach, VA 23452   804/468-3130

Safety-Zone   Free catalog
340 Poplar Street   800/638-6366
Hanover, PA 17333-0028

SelfCare Catalog   Free catalog
349 Healdsburg Avenue   800/345-3371
Healdsburg, CA 95448

Wholesale/Retail Health Appliances

Acme Equipment   Free catalog
1024 Concert Avenue   800/201-0706
Spring Hill, FL 34609

Health and Environment-Related Products

The Ecology Box   Free catalog
P.O. Box 277   800/735-1371
Clinton, MI 49236

Environmentally Safe Products

The Compassionate Consumer, Inc.   Free catalog
(Cruelty Free Products)   516/359-3983
P.O. Box 27
Jericho, NY 11753

Environmentally Safe
Natural Products for Baby

Baby Basics   Free catalog
P.O. Box 224   800/778-3887
East Rockaway, NY 11518

Food and Products For Pets

Halo, Purely For Pets   Free catalog
(Natural Pet Care Products for Dogs,   and animal
Cats, and Birds)   care booklet
3438 East Lake Road—#14   800/426-4256
Palm Harbor, FL 34685

The Natural Pet Care Co.   Free catalog
8050 Lake City Way   800/962-8266
Seattle, WA 98115   206/522-1667

Harbingers of a New Age   Free catalog
717 East Missoula Avenue   800/884-6262
Troy, MT 59935-9609

Cornucopia Natural Pet Products   Free catalog
229 Wall Street   800/PET-8280
Huntington, NY 11743   516/427-7479

Natural Foods

Jaffe Bros. Inc.   Free catalog
P.O. Box 636—Dept. JL   619/749-1133
Valley Center, CA 92082-0636

Gold Mine Natural Food Co.   Free catalog
3419 Hancock Street   800/475-FOOD
San Diego, CA 92110

Clear Eye Natural Foods   Free catalog
302 Rt. 89 South   800/724-2233
Savannah, NY 13146-9711

Fat Free Foods

Fatwise $1 for Catalog
P.O. Box 25—Dept. 308 800/773-8822
Colonia, NJ 07067-0025

Specialty Cookware and Macrobiotic Foods

Mountain Ark Trading Co. Free catalog
P.O. Box 3170 800/643-8909
Fayetteville, AR 72702

Vitamins, Nutritional Supplements, and More

Freeda Vitamins* Free catalog
36 East 41st Street 800/777-3737
New York, NY 10017 212/685-4980
*All products are 100% kosher, yeast-free, vegetarian, and
Feingold-approved for hyperactive children.

Bio-Defense Nutritionals Free catalog
12056 Mt. Vernon Avenue—#201 800/669-9205
Grand Terrace, CA 92313

Future Med Inc. Free catalog
8321 E. Evans Road—#102 800/800-8849
Scottsdale, AZ 85260

Star Professional Pharmaceuticals Free catalog
1500 New Horizons Boulevard 800/274-6400
Amityville, NY 11701

L&H Vitamins Free catalog
32–33 47th Avenue 800/221-1152
Long Island City, NY 11101

Puritan's Pride Free catalog
1233 Montauk Highway 800/645-1030
P.O. Box 9001
Oakdale, NY 11769-9001

Willard Water and More

Dakota Providers   Free catalog
P.O. Box 8023   800/447-4793
Fargo, ND 58109

Gems and New-Age Products and Gifts

Crystal Gardens   Free catalog
21 Greenwich Avenue   212/727-0692
New York, NY 10014

The Nature Company   Free catalog
P.O. Box 188   800/227-1114
Florence, KY 41022

Pacific Spirit   Free catalog
1334 Pacific Avenue   800/634-9057
Forest Grove, OR 97116

Red Rose Collection   Free catalog
P.O. Box 280140   800/220-ROSE
San Francisco, CA 94128-0140

Aromatherapy Products and More

Aroma Vera   Free catalog
5901 Rodeo Road   800/669-9514
Los Angeles, CA 90016   310/280-0407

Oshadhi   Free catalog
P.O. Box 824   501/636-0579
Rogers, AR 72757

Aromaland   Free catalog
Rt. 20—Box 29AL   800/933-5267
Santa Fe, NM 87501

Flower Essence Services   Free catalog
P.O. Box 1769   800/548-0075
Nevada City, CA 95959   916/265-0258

Health-Related Travel Products and More

Magellan's   Free catalog
(Essentials for the Traveler)   800/962-4943
Box 5485
Santa Barbara, CA 93150-5485

Natural Fiber Clothes

Garnet Hill   Free catalog
262 Main Street   800/622-6216
Franconia, NH 03580

The Cotton Place   Free catalog
P.O. Box 7715   800/451-8866
Waco, TX 76714

Reflections Organic, Inc.   Free catalog
Rt. 2—Box 24P40   800/852-9273
Trinity, TX 75862   409/594-9019

Gifts from Your Government

For a free catalog of hundreds of free and low-cost federal publications of consumer interest (e.g., Weight Control; Health, Food, and Nutrition; Exercise; Safety) write to:

Consumer Information Center
Pueblo, CO 81009

Services

There are many health-related services that most people do not know about. Here are some of the ones we know about and want to share with you.

Product Safety
The U.S. Consumer Product Safety Commission has an around-the-clock hotline with information on harmful products. With paper and pencil in hand, call: 800/638-2772; Maryland residents call: 800/492-8104

Check Up on Specialists
The American Board of Medical Specialties has a toll-free number for you to call when you want to make sure that a "specialist" is just that. When you call, give them the doctor's name and they will tell you whether the doctor is listed in a specialty and the year of certification. Call weekdays, between 9 A.M.–6 P.M. EST—800/776-CERT

Naturopath Referral Service
To locate a naturopathic physician in the U.S., send $5.00 for the AANP National Referral Directory and two information brochures to:

American Association of Naturopathic Physicians
2366 Eastlake Avenue E.—#322
Seattle, WA 98102

Self-Help Support Groups
There are approximately 500,000 support groups throughout the country, helping nurture an estimated fifteen million people. The process of sharing with others who have similar physical or mental health problems can help ease those problems and offer a support system that includes information on the most current medical research. To find local support groups in your area, write to or call:

National Self-Help Clearing House   212/354-8525
CUNY Graduate Center
25 West 43rd Street—Suite 620
New York, NY 10036

Ailment Information Including Holistic Alternatives
LaVerne and Steve Ross are cofounders of the World Research Foundation. They have an incredible service. For a nominal fee, they will do a search (which includes 5,000 international medical journals) and provide you with the newest holistic and conventional treatments and diagnostic techniques on most any condition. The Foundation's library of more than 10,000 books, periodicals, and research reports is available to the public free of charge. Write or call:

World Research Foundation   800/WRF-HELP
15300 Ventura Boulevard—Suite 405   818/907-5483
Sherman Oaks, CA 91403

International Travelers' Health Information
The National Centers for Disease Control has a hotline that provides information on food and water precautions, vaccinations, and other facts relevant to international travel. With pencil and paper in hand, call: 404/332-4559

Recommended Reading

As of this writing, all of these wonderful books are in print. If they're not in your local book stores, ask the store manager to order them for you, or call the publisher and order directly. (We've provided publisher's phone numbers.)

Spontaneous Healing by Andrew Weil, M.D. How to discover and enhance your body's natural ability to maintain and heal itself. (Alfred A. Knopf, Inc.; 800/733-3000)

The Family Herbal by Barbara & Peter Theiss. A guide to natural health care for yourself and your children. (Healing Arts Press; 802/767-3174)

Natural Alternatives to Antibiotics by Ray C. Wunderlich, Jr., M.D. Antibiotic overuse is now an epidemic, creating deadly new strains of drug-resistant bacteria. Dr. Wunderlich discusses a wide range of safe remedies that work with your body to fight illness. (Keats Publishing, Inc.; 800/858-7014, ext. 18)

Between Heaven and Earth by Harriet Beinfield L.Ac. and Efrem Korngold, L.Ac., OMD. A guide to Chinese medicine. (Ballantine Books; 800/733-3000)

Beating Alzheimer's by Tom Warren. The remarkable story of how one man reversed the devastating symptoms of Alzheimer's Disease. (Avery Publishing; 800/548-5757)

Royden Brown's *Bee Hive Product Bible.* A complete guide to bee pollen, propolis, honey, and royal jelly for health, vitality, and beauty. (Avery Publishing; 800/548-5757)

500 Fat-Free Recipes by Sarah Schlesinger. A complete guide to reducing the fat in your diet. Delicious and healthful recipes. (Villard Books; 800/733-3000)

Fat Free & Ultra Lowfat Recipes by Doris Cross. Combines recipes for optimum health with delicious taste. (Prima Publishing; 800/632-8676)

Lick the Sugar Habit by Nancy Appleton, Ph.D. Sugar addiction upsets your whole body chemistry. This book tells you how to overcome the addiction. (Avery Publishing; 800/548-5757)

Doctor, What Should I Eat? by Isadore Rosenfeld, M.D. Nutrition prescriptions for ailments in which diet can really make a difference. (Random House; 800/733-3000)

Eat More, Weigh Less by Dean Ornish, M.D. Dr. Ornish's life choice program for losing weight safely while eating abundantly. (HarperCollins; 800/331-3761)

Kombucha Phenomenon—The Tea Mushroom Handbook by Betsy Pryor & Sanford Holst. Everything you ever wanted to know about the *health tonic* that's sweeping America. (Sierra Sunrise Books, 14622 Ventura Blvd., Suite 800, Sherman Oaks, CA 91403)

The Complete Book of Dental Remedies by Flora Parsa-Stay D.D.S. A guide to safe and effective relief from the most common dental problems using homeopathy, nutritional supplements, herbs, and conventional dental care. (Avery Publishing; 800/548-5757)

Stop Aging Now by Jean Carper. The ultimate plan for staying young and reversing the aging process. (HarperCollins; 800/331-3761)

Inner Peace—Outer Beauty by Michelle Dominique Leight. Natural Japanese health and beauty secrets revealed. (A Citadel Press Book published by Carol Publishing Group; 800/447-BOOK)

Smart Medicine for Menopause by Sandra Cabot, M.D. A no-nonsense guide to using H.R.T., herbs, vitamins, foods, and natural supplements to ease the discomfort of menopause. (Avery Publishing; 800/548-5757)

Sharks Don't Get Cancer by Dr. I. William Lane and Linda Comac. A remarkable new breakthrough in the prevention and treatment of cancer and other degenerative diseases. (Avery Publishing; 800/548-5757)

Nontoxic, Natural & Earthwise by Debra Lynn Dadd. How to protect yourself and your family from harmful products and live in harmony with the Earth. (Jeremy P. Tarcher, Inc.; 800/631-8571)

Vegetarian Cats & Dogs by James A. Peden. A classic on vegetarian companion animals. Find answers to your questions in this well-researched book. (Harbingers of a New Age; 800/884-6262)

Your Own Perfect Medicine by Martha M. Christy. The incredible proven natural miracle cure that medical science has never revealed. A fascinating comprehensive book of the mainstream medical uses of urine therapy, proving its ability to cure an extraordinary number of illnesses. (Future Med Inc.; 800/800-8849)

Peace, Love & Healing—Bodymind Communication and the Path to Self-Healing: An Exploration by Dr. Bernie S. Siegel. (HarperCollins; 800/331-3761)

Love, Medicine & Miracles—Self Healing from a Surgeon's Experience with Exceptional Patients by Dr. Bernie S. Siegel. (HarperCollins; 800/331-3761)

Healing Into Immortality: A New Spiritual Medicine of Stories and Imaging by Gerald Epstein. (Bantam Books; 800/223-5780)

A Cozy Book of Herbal Teas by Mindy Toomay. Recipes, remedies, and folk wisdom. (Prima Publishing; 800/632-8676)

The Healing Power of Herbs by Michael T. Murray ND. The enlightened person's guide to the wonders of medicinal plants. (Prima Publishing; 800/632-8676)

Chicken Soup & Other Folk Remedies by Joan Wilen & Lydia Wilen. (Fawcett Columbine; 800/733-3000)

More Chicken Soup & Other Folk Remedies by Joan Wilen & Lydia Wilen. (Fawcett Columbine; 800/733-3000)

Dr. Whitaker's Guide to Natural Healing by Julian Whitaker, M.D. This book helps arm you with the information you need to trigger the body's tremendous power to heal itself. (Prima Publishing; 800/632-8676)

Encyclopedia of Natural Medicine by Michael Murray, ND and Joseph Pizzorno, ND. In an easy-to-understand manner, this book explains the principles of natural medicine and outlines their application through the safe and effective use of herbs, vitamins, minerals, diet, and nutrition. (Prima Publishing; 800/632-8676)

Alternative Medicine: The Definitive Guide compiled by The Burton Goldberg Group. This very big and exceptional book, with input by over 400 leading alternative health professionals, sharing their effective therapies and affordable self-help cures, is well worth the cover price. (Future Medicine Publishing; for information call: 800/990-9499, to place an order call: 800/637-7524)

Index

Dandelion, 216, 276; and diabetes, 84
—tea: for arthritis, 18; for gout, 24; for mastitis, 179; to reduce swelling, 40
Dandruff, 113–14
Deafness, prevention of, 91
Decongestants, 74
Dehydration, 11–12, 66, 86
Dentures, 276
Deodorants, 38–39, 152
Depression, 79–82, 180
Desserts, and gout, 23
Diabetes, 83–85, 173
Diaper rash, 163
Diaries, 80–81, 260–61
Diarrhea, 86–88, 173; in infants, 163–64; in pets, 198, 203
Diet: and alcoholism, 8; and allergies, 120–21; and appendicitis, 14; and arteriosclerosis, 140; and arthritis, 19–20; and baldness, 116; and blood pressure, 34–35; and canker sores, 48; and cold sores, 62; and colic in infants, 162; and constipation, 69; diabetes and, 83–84; and diarrhea, 86; and fatigue, 99–100; and fingernail problems, 108; and gallbladder, 111–12; and gout, 23; and hearing loss, 91; and herpes genitalis, 145–46; and hyperactivity in children, 53–54; and itching skin, 169; natural foods, 296; of pets, 199, 201–202, 205–206; and sleepiness, 99; and stress, 263; and ulcers, 278
Dill seed tea, 148, 155, 214, 277; for colicky baby, 162
Dill tea, 73, 153, 246
Dirty dishes, and insomnia, 246
Dogs, treatments for, 198–205
Dolomite, 228
Dong quai, 185, 186–87, 226
Douches, for vaginitis, 286
Dreams, bad, in children, 51
Dried fruits, 169

Driving, drinking and, 10
Drowsiness, 100
Drunkenness, prevention of, 9
Dry-food worm repellent, 168
Dry mouth, 277
Dry skin, 239–40; in dogs, 205
Dulse, for broken bones, 40
Dusting, before vacuuming, 151

E, vitamin, 187; and age spots, 237; for mastitis, 179; for sciatica, 221; for varicose veins, 288
—oil, 62, 78, 236; for corns, 105; for cradle cap, 163; for ear mites, 198; for fingernails, 108; for genital warts, 291; for hemorrhoids, 143; for herpes genitalis, 145; for insect stings, 165; for pet wounds, 205; and poison ivy, 210; and ringworm, 218; for shingles, 231; for toenail fungus, 102; for warts, 289
Ear care, for dogs, 203
Ear mites, 198
Ears, 89–93; pierced, 121
Eating alone, 57
Echinacea, 134
Eczema, 238–39
Egg white, 55, 96, 157, 228, 240; baking soda and, for burns, 46; for hemorrhoids, 144; for sprains, 191
Egg yolk: facial conditioner, 239–40; shampoo, 116
Eggplant, 19, 60, 240, 289
Eggs, 77, 120, 132–33; human, 161, 227; silver and, for bruises, 42
Eilat stone, 31
Elderflower tea, 231
Electrolytes, 86
Emotions, 6–7, 28, 35, 48, 207
Endive, 216
Environment, sleep, 245
Environment-related products, 305–306
Epsom salts, for gallstones, 111
Estrogen, and depression, 80

Hot spices, as aphrodisiac, 224
Hot weather, 134, 136
House fly repellents, 166–67
Household problems, 150–52
Humidity, for dry coughs, 75
Hyperactivity in children, 53–54
Hyssop, 120

Ice, 134; for black eyes, 42–43; for
    cold sores, 61; for diarrhea, 87;
    for hiccups, 148; for insect
    stings, 165; for migraine, 128;
    for motion sickness, 189; for
    nausea, 159; for pimples, 241;
    for sinus, 232; for sprains, 191;
    for tired feet, 103
ICE-PILLO, 128, 129
Immune system, 134, 172
Impotence, 173, 224–26
Incontinence, 173
Indigestion, 153–60, 173, 249
Infants, 161–64; products for, 306
Infertility, 227–28
Ingrown toenails, 103
Insects, 165–68
Insomnia, 246, 249
Intuition, in gem therapy, 3–4
Iodine, 296
Iron: dietary, 48, 108, 169; from
    cookware, 132
Itching, 83, 169–70; of ears, 91;
    vaginal, 286

Jade, 40–41
Jade plant, and cataracts, 96–97
Jalapeño peppers, 140
Jasmine, 221, 223
Jerusalem artichokes, 84
Jewelweed, 209
Jock itch, 170
Jojoba oil, 90
Jokes, for health, 299–301

K, vitamin, and broken bones,
    40
Kale, 116, 216
Kelp, 17–18, 36, 141, 296
Kidneys, 173, 281–84
Kiwi, 35, 153
Knees, bruised, 44

Kombucha Tea Mushroom,
    171–77
Kosher salt, for cold feet, 105

Lady's mantle tea, 295
Lamb, 145
Lamb's wool, 32
Lameness, in dogs, 203
Laryngitis, 256–57
Laughter, 72; healing, 299–301
Lavender, 120, 168, 223
Lead, from ceramics, 132
Lecithin, 60, 221, 296
Leek juice, for shingles, 230
Legs: cramps, 192–93; shaving of,
    134
Legumes, 84, 224
Lemon oil, 100
Lemons, 137, 138, 168, 199, 272;
    for boils, 237; for chapped
    hands, 238; for constipation, 70;
    for coughs, 73; for dandruff,
    114; for feet, 104, 105–106; hair
    spray, 116; hangover cure, 11;
    for hemorrhoids, 143; for
    hiccups, 148; for motion
    sickness, 190; for neuralgia, 194;
    for sore throat, 254; for
    wrinkles, 244
Lentils, 145
Lettuce, 157, 216
Lice, 54
Lifting, and back problems, 30
Lima beans, 145, 252
Limbic system, 2
Lime juice, 164, 270
Listerine, for plantar warts, 291
Liver spots. See Age spots
L-lysine, 62, 145–46
Long-term memory, 182
Loss of hair, 113, 116–17
Low-fat diets, infants and, 164
Lyme tick repellent, 168

Macrobiotic foods, 307
Magnesium, 80, 100; and calcium,
    192
Magnolia bark tea, 252
Makeup remover, 241
Malachite, 193

Mango, 153
Marjoram tea, 252
Masks, to prevent hay fever, 118
Massage: for hiccups, 148; for
    neuralgia, 194; for sciatica, 221;
    for stomach upset, 154; for
    tension headaches, 124
Mastitis, 178–79
Mayonnaise, hair conditioner, 115
Meat, 112; and gout, 23
Meat tenderizer, for stings, 165
Medication, and memory loss, 180
Meditation, 264
Melatonin, 222
Melons, 71, 120
Memory, 173, 180–83
Men: constipation remedy, 70;
    housework by, 135; infertility
    remedies, 228; smoking, 249
Menopause, 173, 184–85
Menstruation, 11, 186–88
Mental exercises, 181
Metal removers, 136
Microwaving, 136
Migraine headaches, 127–29
Milk, 120, 169, 206–207, 264, 276
Millet, for tired feet, 103
Mineral oil, for swimmer's ear, 90
Minor injuries, 54; cuts, 77
Mint, 167, 205, 257
Miscarriage, 212; smoking and,
    227, 249
Miso, 137
Mittens, 131
Moisturizers, for skin, 241
Molasses, for eczema, 238
Months, best for sex, 222
Moon phases, 136; and diabetes,
    84
Morning coughs, 75
Morning headaches, 125
Morning sickness, 213–14
Morning stiffness, to prevent, 21
Mosquito repellents, 166–67
Moth repellents, 168
Mothballs, to repel cats, 206
Motion sickness, 189–90, 214
Mouth problems, 270–77; pepper
    burns, 46–47
Mucus, to clear, 26–27

Mud, for insect stings, 165
Mugwort tea, and poison ivy, 210
Multiple sclerosis, 173
Muscle pains, 191–93
Muscle spasms, in feet, 103
Mushroom, Kombucha Tea,
    171–77
Mushrooms, 23, 46, 108, 236, 252
Music, healing, 261, 301
Musical instruments, for asthma,
    26
Mustard, 49, 104–105, 143, 156,
    270; to bring on period, 187
Mustard greens, 216, 276
Mustard seeds, for constipation,
    69
Myrrh, 49, 79; for gums, 275, 276
Myrtillin, 84

Nail polish, 61, 109
Natural foods, 296, 306
Natural remedies for constipation,
    69–72
Nausea, 157–59
Neck, stiff, 259
Negative thoughts, 299
Neroli, 141
Nervousness, 260–66; coughs, 76
Nettles, 119; tea, for acne, 236
Neuralgia, 194–95
Neuritis, 194
Neuropathy, 194
New Age products, 308
Newspaper ink, for nausea, 159,
    190
Nickel, allergy to, 121
Night sweats, 184
Night vision, 97
Nightmares, 247; in children, 51
Nightshade foods, 19
Nose: runny, 66; stuffy, 66, 120
Nosebleed, 196–97
Nutmeg, 148, 158
Nuts, 23, 62, 100, 120, 121, 145

Oat bran, for constipation, 69
Oatmeal, 23, 210, 268
Oats, and cholesterol, 59
Oatstraw baths for broken bones,
    40

Potato water, to clean silver, 135
Potatoes, 19, 35, 62, 86, 145; for
    eyestrain, 95; for frigidity, 227;
    for neuralgia, 195; for upset
    stomach, 153
—raw: for bruises, 43; for eczema,
    238; for eyes, 243, 268
Poultices, 5; bay leaf, for coughs,
    74–75; for bruises, 43; for
    burns, 46; for chest congestion
    in infants, 161; dandelion, to
    reduce swelling, 40; for eyes,
    95, 243, 268; for hemorrhoids,
    144; horseradish, for headaches,
    123; for mastitis, 178–79; for
    neuralgia, 194, 195; radish, for
    stiff neck, 259; for sciatica, 220;
    for varicose ulcers, 288; yarrow,
    for toothache, 271
Poultry, and gout, 23
Prayer, for heart health, 142
Pregnancy, 5, 212–15; and
    migraine, 129; pennyroyal oil
    and, 199
Premenstrual syndrome (PMS),
    173, 186–87
Preparation of herbs, 4–6
Preservatives, and allergies, 121
Pressure-point therapy for motion
    sickness, 189–90
Printers' ink, smell of, 159, 190
Problem-solving, 137
Prostate problems, 173, 216–17
Prunes, 70–71, 216
Psoriasis, 173, 242–43
Psychological impotence, 224–25
Psyllium, 71–72; tea for weight
    control, 295
Puffy eyes, potato for, 243
Pumpernickel, 145
Pumpkin, for insomnia, 246
Pumpkin seeds, 108, 236; for
    constipation, 70; for impotence,
    226; for prostate health, 216
Pygeum Africanum extract, 217

Radioactivity, to remove, 137
Radishes, 251; for burns, 46; as
    deodorant, 38; juice, for hang-
    overs, 9; for stiff neck, 259

Ragweed, 120
Raisins, 108, 252, 272; and gin for
    arthritis, 15–16
Raspberries, 116
Raspberry leaf tea, 153, 187–88;
    for pregnant women, 212–13
Rectal itching, 169–70
Red clover tea, 119
Red wine, 127; for cold sores, 62
Reflexology: for earaches, 90; for
    hemorrhoids, 144; for nausea,
    159; for sinus congestion, 233;
    for stomach upset, 154; for
    stress, 264
Resources, 303–309
Rheumatism. See Arthritis
Rhodochrosite, 27, 164, 264
Rice, brown, 23
Rice bran, 283
Ringing in ears, 91–92
Rings, to remove from fingers, 138
Ringworm, 218–19
Romaine lettuce, 210
Rosa gallica, 71
Rose, 223
Rose quartz, for pets, 201
Rosemary, 140–41; oil, 167; tea,
    115, 182, 246
Rosin, for gallstones, 111
Royal jelly, 228
Ruby, 223
Rumbling stomach, 159–60
Runny nose, 66
Rutabagas, and cholesterol, 59

SAD. See Seasonal Affective
    Disorder
Safflower oil, 205
Sage tea, 117, 153, 155; for
    laryngitis, 257; for memory,
    182; and miscarriage, 212
Salads, 70, 138
Salicylate, 29; and tinnitus, 91
Salmon, 276
Salmonella, to avoid, 132–33
Salt, 36, 138–39; and arthritis,
    19–20; for itching, 169; for
    poison ivy, 208–209; to remove
    pesticides, 137; for sore throat,
    254; for sprains, 191

Strep throat, 256
Stress, 48, 173, 260–66; and
    infertility, 227
Stretch marks, 212
String beans, 281–82
Stuffy nose, 120
Styptic pencil, 49
Subconscious, 2
Sugar, 120; and freckles, 240; and
    insects, 166; massage for bruise,
    42; and yeast infection, 286
Sugarless gum, and plaque, 273
Sugilite, 110, 146
Sulfur, 136; and baldness, 116
Suma, 185, 188
Sunburn, 267–69
Sunflower seeds, 35, 108, 224,
    236, 251; for energy, 99
Sunlight: and depression, 81; and
    sex, 222
Supplements, nutritional, 307
Sweet basil, 167
Sweet potatoes, 70, 136, 216, 252
Sweets, substitutes for, 295
Swelling, to reduce, 40, 43–44
Swimmers: ear infections, 90–91;
    leg cramps, 193
Swiss chard, 216
Swiss cheese, 276
Synthetic fabrics, 39

Tabasco sauce, 26, 66
Talking in sleep, 247
Tangerine juice, hangover remedy,
    12
Tansy, 167
Tape, to remove splinters, 258
Tartar, to prevent, 275
Tea: angelica, for alcoholism, 8;
    bayberry, for constipation, 70;
    borage, for grief, 80; burdock
    root, for psoriasis, 243;
    camomile, for gallbladder, 111;
    catnip, for ulcers, 278–79;
    celery, for sciatica, 221; cleaning
    with, 135; for coughs, 73, 74,
    75; dandelion, to reduce
    swelling, 40; for eyestrain,
    94–95; fennel, as deodorant,
    38–39; elderflower, for shingles,

231; for hair, 115; hawthorn
    berry, 35–36, 142; for heart
    palpitations, 140–41;
    horehound, for sore throat, 255;
    for impotence, 226; to increase
    breast milk, 214; for insomnia,
    246; for kidneys, 282, 283; for
    laryngitis, 257; for mastitis,
    178–79; for memory, 182; for
    morning sickness, 214; nettle,
    for acne, 236; pennyroyal, for
    fleas, 199; to prevent allergies,
    119; to prevent plaque, 273; for
    prostate health, 217; raspberry,
    for women, 187–88, 212–13;
    sesame seed, for toothache, 271;
    for sinus congestion, 232; for
    smelly feet, 106; to stop
    smoking, 252; for stress,
    261–62; for weight control, 295
—dill seed: for colicky baby, 162;
    for hiccups, 148
—fenugreek seed: for asthma,
    26–27; for ringing in ears, 92
—ginger root: for colds, 65–66; for
    cough with phlegm, 75; for
    hangovers, 12
—herbal, 5, 135; for arthritis, 18;
    and diabetes, 84; for gas pains,
    155; for gout, 24; for upset
    stomach, 153
—oatstraw: for broken bones, 40;
    for varicose veins, 288
—sage: for hair, 117; to avoid
    miscarriage, 212
—yarrow: for back problems, 29;
    for menstrual problems, 187; to
    prevent nosebleed, 197
Tea, Kombucha Mushroom,
    171–77
Tea bags: for smelly feet, 106; for
    sunburned eyes, 268
Tea leaves, to stop bleeding, 77
Tea tree oil, 54
Teeth, problems with, 54–55, 164,
    270–77
Telephone, 30; and laryngitis, 256
Television, and bed-wetting, 52
Temporal headaches, 126–27
Tender feet, to toughen, 104

330 · INDEX